COMPUTATIONAL MATHEMATICS AND ANALYSIS

MODELS AND METHODS FOR SUPPORTING DECISION-MAKING IN HUMAN HEALTH AND ENVIRONMENT PROTECTION

COMPUTATIONAL MATHEMATICS AND ANALYSIS

Additional books in this series can be found on Nova's website under the Series tab.

Additional e-books in this series can be found on Nova's website under the eBooks tab.

COMPUTATIONAL MATHEMATICS AND ANALYSIS

MODELS AND METHODS FOR SUPPORTING DECISION-MAKING IN HUMAN HEALTH AND ENVIRONMENT PROTECTION

CARLOS N. BOUZA
FLÁVIO L. DE MELLO
AND
MARCOS NEGREIROS
EDITORS

nova publishers
New York

Library of Congress Cataloging-in-Publication Data
Names: Bouza, Carlos N., editor. | Mello, Flávio L. de, editor. | Negreiros, Marcos, editor.
Title: Models and methods for supporting decision-making in human health and environment protection / editors, Carlos N. Bouza, Flávio L. de Mello and Marcos Negreiros (Facultad de Matematica y Computacion, Universidad de La Habana, Cuba, and others).
Description: Hauppauge, New York : Nova Science Publisher's, Inc., [2016] | Series: Computational mathematics and analysis | Includes index.
Identifiers: LCCN 2016014508 (print) | LCCN 2016023429 (ebook) | ISBN 9781634851732 (hardcover) | ISBN 9781634852029 (ebook) | ISBN 9781634852029 ()
Subjects: LCSH: Environmental health--Decision making.
Classification: LCC RA566 .M63 2016 (print) | LCC RA566 (ebook) | DDC 362.1--dc23
LC record available at https://lccn.loc.gov/2016014508

Published by Nova Science Publishers, Inc. † New York

CONTENTS

PREFACE

This book aims to present models and methods for objective analysis associated to human health and environment protection. The content deals mainly with specific models based on statistics, operational research and mathematical logic, as well as the need for developing efficient software. Despite the existence of powerful computing capacity, the availability of commercial packages capable to deal with the particular needs of hospitals, health institutions and environmental phenomena it is not very common. The mainstream research and development usually is strict to high-level management or to the most profitable thematic areas.

Other books have approached the themes covered in this volume. However, they do not include simultaneously statistics, operations research, and computing aspects needed for developing efficient decision support procedures. Under this perspective, the concept behind the organization of this work is to provide a reference for exploring models, explaining features and interpreting aspects in details as well as allowing training the readers to fit them in practice.

This collection aims to provide an overall view of methodological aspects that make all the presented approaches and models feasible and reproducible by the reader, thus familiarizing he or she with contemporary efforts for modeling and illustrating their use in practice. The book not only completely describes the models but also presents real applications, based on the authors' experience. Features and interconnections are emphasized in the different chapters through analysis discussion, interpretation, and implementation. We believe that the discussions and interpretations pervading the contents of the book will contribute to readers' improvement.

The model-based analysis, the software procedures and the real study cases emphasize the relevance of both theoretical and practical expertise. The readership target groups are graduate students or researchers in statistics, operations research, and computing; professionals dealing with psychometric, social, biomedical, and pedagogical sciences; practitioners.

The first five chapters address statistic issues applied to human health and environment protection. The next four chapters concern the use of mathematical logic to improve modelling and decision-making. The last five chapters deal with operational research. Moreover, readers interested in more advanced topics will obtain references for consulting contemporary literature on several themes.

This initiative is part of the Project CAPES-MES-CUBA 209/13, which promotes joint research between Cuban and Brazilian specialists, aiming to develop theoretical and practical aspects of modeling by providing mathematical models and efficient software. This cooperation is designed for dealing with medical and environmental issues. Some manuscripts are based on presentations in the workshop *Experiences in Image Processing, Decision Support and Information Systems for Health Decision*, held in Aracati – Brazil, and in the *11th International Workshop on Operations Research* developed in La Habana – Cuba. Cuban and Brazilian researchers shared their experiences in these workshops. During these two events, it became evident the necessity for publishing this book in order to spread the proposed solution for the incoming problems. The editorial board was selected from operations research, statistics and computing experts.

We thank CAPES, Coppetec Foundation Project Poli 19.257, and PNCB Modelos Matemáticos para el Estudio de Medio Ambiente, Salud y Desarrollo Humano for supporting this cooperation. We also thank Nova Publishers for the interest in this project and the constant attention in its development.

The Editors

In: Models and Methods for Supporting Decision-Making … ISBN: 978-1-63485-173-2
Editors: Carlos N. Bouza, Flávio L. de Mello et al.

Chapter 1

CALCULATING CHARACTERIZATION OF MONOPSONIC DEGREE IN THE RECYCLED SOLID WASTE MARKET IN METROPOLITAN REGIONS OF BRAZIL

Rilton Gonçalo Bonfim Primo[1,*] and José Félix García Rodríguez[2,†]
[1]Centro de Estudios por la Amistad de Latinoamérica, Asia y África, Brazil
[2]Departamento de Ciencias Económicas y Administrativas,
Universidad Juárez Autónoma de Tabasco, Villahermosa, TAB, Mexico

ABSTRACT

The goal of this essay is to encourage and make an aport to calculate the characterization of monopsony in the market of recycled solid waste in metropolitan regions of Brazil. This was done by estimating the corresponding deviation between price and added value, circumstantially and structurally privileging the links in the chain of reverse logistics of residue, from the lone scavenger to the industry. We will make a theoretical approach of the social significance of concentrated markets. This work presents a tool to calculate the degree of monopsonization, which is a first step towards Fair Trade. It also refers to an efficient experimentation in the Northeast of Brazil.

Keywords: reverse logistics, fair trade, mathematical foundations, practical method with excel

---

* Rilton Gonçalo Bonfim Primo: Rua Areal de Baixo, nº 136, apto. 414, Largo 2 de Julho, Salvador, Bahia, Brasil. CEP 40060-210. E-mail: riltonprimo@hotmail.com.
† José Félix García Rodríguez: Carrillo Puerto, nº 272, Colonia Carrizal, CP 86108, Vilhermosa, Tabasco, México. E-mail: jfgr55@hotmail.com.

INTRODUCTION

Various forms of self-employment have arisen on the five continents: services, small production studios, workshops, mobile improvised facilities and many other kinds. This has taken place even inside the value chain of the sector of recycled solid waste, in which the work forms characterize the fragility and precariousness of their relations with the market.

The first step to a *Project to Calculate the Characterization of Monopsonic Degree* is justified on account of the multilateral fight of the civil society and the public authorities against the inefficient distribution-allocation, which is a result of the concentration. This situation has a strong theoretical and quantifiable basis:

> The trend toward concentration, that created situations of virtual monopoly in certain branches, provoked reversed reactions in defense of the public interest, such as the antitrust laws of the end of the last century. Once the door to monopoly was closed, it was necessary to develop subtler coordination methods. The oligopoly [and oligopsony] is the culmination of this evolution: it allows a small group of large firms to create barriers for the entrance of others in a sector of economic activity and to co-manage the prices of certain products, preserving, however, financial, technological and administrative autonomy. The price management creates a relative advantage for the companies that innovate more, both in productive processes and in the introduction of new products in a given sector. Differently from the traditional competition of prices (which translates into reduction of profits, financial weakening, closed factories or, in the case of a monopoly, increase in prices and reduction of demand), the world of the oligopolies looks more like [...] a sport to which only champions have access [1].

The aim of this chapter is to contribute to the process of consistent definition of values for products or services – from the dialogical, transparent and effective participation of all the actors involved in its composition – resulting in a trade that provides equitable distribution of gains in the productive chain, according to article #2 of the Decree n. 7.358. This law is a new and advanced instrument to solidarity.

The issue of the relative weakness of recyclers at a highly concentrated market is impressive. Only a few actors dictate prices and conditions. It is not a regional exception, but a conflict of indigence against opulence in very poor regions.

> The industries are the most benefited by the entire process of recycling garbage in Brazil and in the world, precisely because they are highly concentrated, representing a model of oligopsony, when a small number of companies consumes the recyclable materials and imposes the conditions and prices to the gatherers and cooperatives, making them the hostages of the exploitation of the informal economy by the formal one. This is the sad situation of the agents that work with garbage in our country. Regarding cooperatives/associations or autonomous gatherers, the exploitation happens in all levels of the productive and reproductive sequence of recycling. Under these conditions, the recycling itself does not represent a cost-effective alternative and much less an environmental one; it only shortly smothers the social pressures on the unemployment of the excluded ones and provides a gain for the industries, through the reduction of their costs. They use the scraps, the great "lords of garbage," and control the market of recycled products [2].

Rigorously, it is not possible to calculate a rate of exploitation of the scavengers[1], because it is calculated based on the salary. In most cases, they do not have salary.

> The scavenger would also be associated with the term exploitation. According to the literature, they would be exploited by other more articulated sectors of the chain […], due to the very structure of the recycling market and to the sectors that dominate it – intermediaries and industry -, the formation of informal oligopsonies is common, which leads to a control of the price paid for the material [4].

The discussion of *Fair Trade* today is renewed with technical and empirical reviews:

> The issue of marketing is quite complex and involves several aspects that deserve special attention, once considered the limit for the improvement of the conditions of marketing cooperatives. Even if they have gained some power of negotiation of prices, the recycling market […] is an oligopsony. For example, there is only a small number of purchasers: "Without competition, a product such as the recyclable material separated from the source [or not] is sold at a price that the oligopsony wants to pay, which keeps the cost of reverse flow extremely cheap." The power of the industry is evident in the analysis […] that attributes to this segment of the value chain up to 75% of total possible gains provided by recycling [5].

The researcher R. Smith, in his *Unequal Trade and Industrialization in the Northeast*, explained that contemporaneously "the unequal exchange is focused as the non-equivalent exchange of quantities of work (or value)" and it is enclosed into the free trade. There are those economists "that admit the non-equivalence in trade as a result of a mismatch in transitional competition, since it does not lose the referential of equilibrium." And there are "those who admit to non-transience of deviation in market prices in relation to the prices of production. The oligopolistic capitalism determines the permanent nature of this deviation" [6]. This is precisely the scenario of the concentrated sector.

> In the cycle of recyclable materials, recycling companies located on the upper circuit use a technology of relatively high level of expertise, usually capital intensive and originating from advanced countries. Thus, the activities of the upper circuit tend to concentrate power and to control the cycle as a whole. It is important to remember that the market for recyclable is configured, on the demand side, as an oligopsony – few companies have the ability to purchase certain goods -, which further demonstrates the concentration exerted by this upper circuit. In this way, the materials collected by the workers of the lower circuit (which create a situation of "perfect competition" on the supply side) are separated and then sent to the companies. In this process, the material

[1] "In response to the virtual loss of source of income, the path already paved by the gatherers is the collective organization of the sector. The immediate gain to the organized scavenger is related to the terms and conditions of work he finds in cooperatives, as regular working hours, personal protective equipment and sanitary conditions that are more suitable for the performance of his activities. However, the employment bonds are still very weak in most of the cooperatives and associations – only in a minority of the cases these organizations have legal records and are able to obey all of the labor legislation and taxes. In most cases, they do not have enough equipment and knowledge to ensure economic efficiency. The elaboration of public policies focusing on the gatherers will require a more in-depth knowledge of the current situation of organizations of collective work" [3].

will have its value systematically increased as it goes up in the cycle towards the upper circuit [7].

In fact, the markets of solid waste in Brazil are structured as oligopsonies within which a floating number of middlemen who sign frequent price agreements (and other conditions of purchase) proliferate. That not only generates inefficiency in the process of allocation of resources, with reductions in recycled quantities and in the level of society welfare; but also, in particular, they degenerate and begin to diminish the work value of the gatherers, whose income/product is transferred, in a staggered form, to the links above the value chain of the industry. Nationally, the direct demand focuses on traders (middlemen), which are more than half of the supply of waste, followed by the industry (final direct and indirect receiver), with less than 20%. The professor of the *School of Management and Business, of University of Rio Grande*, Maria do Carmo, portrayed the local scenery[2] in Paraná[3]. Among other urban concentrations, the biggest example is São Paulo, with its scenario of Piracicaba, among other thousands of regional examples:

> The marketing of the collected, separated and pressed material by the Cooperative is made by its own recyclers as of a register of buyers. The so-called 'scrap' acquires the materials collected by recyclers and determines prices according to the selling prices (prices at which the materials will be sold to companies that recycle – final companies). On the other hand, in the relationship between the scrap and the final companies, the latter determine the prices. In some cases, this creates a situation of oligopsony [10].

This chapter has two sections, in addition to the conclusions. In the first one, we will review the dynamics of highly concentrated markets from the perspective of the possibilities of abuse and restraint of cartel power. In the second, one of the most used versions of Hirchman Herfindahl-Index (HHI) will be displayed. It is able to estimate the degree of competitiveness of a market. Also in this second section, the HHI will be instrumental for immediate application through Excel, highlighting results of market regulation experiments in northeastern Brazil. Naturally, Excel is a registered product and its license is necessary.

THEORETICAL APPROACH

In *The Economy and the Art of Controversy*, K. Galbraith argued the *unequal exchange*, focusing on the situation of the small farmer[4]. But it is a recurring debate in Political

[2] "Unlike the gatherers, buyers would be well articulated, because the paper trading in the city of Rio de Janeiro is marked by the union of three large middlemen. This union gave rise to Recycling Center of Rio de Janeiro (CRR), - considered the main buyer of material collected by collectors in the city, an oligopsony" [8].

[3] "In the four cities (Paraná) researched, there are no recycling industries installed. All the collected recyclable material is pressed and sent to companies that recycle cardboard, paper, aluminum, glass and plastic. In the case of Paraná, there are five recyclers of paper registered at Cempre (Corporate Commitment to Recycling). If this number is compared to the observation that gathering recyclable material is a reality in more than 200 Paraná municipalities that are related to the Project 'Paran Environmental,' these recyclers are actually forming an oligopsony [9].

[4] "The struggle in the labor market, with its controversy, was the result of primitive inequality in ability to make contracts and the efforts of unions to eliminateit. This inequality is not exclusive to the labor market, nor are the consequences to which it gives rise. A similar problem occurs where there are many people, who are

Economy. In his habilitation thesis, submitted to the Institute *of Economics at the State University of Campinas* (Unicamp), M. Coutinho has resumed the classics, more particularly Adam Smith, in the following sense: "the question of value should refer to the ability that the goods have, in an exchange, to command the labor of others" [13]. But, regardless of whether it is measured by work or by another measurement, the issue is that the value may differ from the price and, in this case, that profits are transferred from the losing party to the winner. In the most recent global stage of mergers/acquisitions, the policies for the prevention of the abuse of power in trade systems, though not restricted to oligopolies (whose action is free), have become commonly used. This has happened in Brazil, and it is opportune to mention it here in a footnote[5]. Also called the "degree of monopoly," the *market power of the company* can be defined in such simple kaleckian terms, that it was once considered tautological, even. Where $K = \frac{p}{u}$, in which p is the *price*, u stands for direct costs and K for the *degree of monopoly*, which changes due to 1) changes in the degree of economic concentration, 2) advertising (and middlemen), 3) The ratio of indirect costs (wages, cost of capital, taxation, etc.) on the direct ones and 4) power of the trade unions/cooperatives. It is worth reminding that the direct costs (u) are determined by the costs with wages (w) and expenditures (both measured per unit of product) with raw materials (m), so that $u = w(1 + j)$, where j is the raw materials quotient by the hourly wage, as (Equation 1).

$$K = \frac{p}{w\left(1+\frac{m}{w}\right)} \tag{1}$$

The influence of the monopoly degree on the formation of prices stands out in this brief argument. Each firm fixes prices by mark-up in a more or less concentrated industry[6]. Low

individually powerless because they are numerous. They make exchanges with some large companies, of much bigger relative strength, precisely because they are few. This is the weakness of the lone worker, who was also characterized, in general, in the situation of the farmer. Typically, the farmer alone does not influence the price of sales or purchases. He lives in a world where, because of the stronger position occupied by other circles of the market, the exercise of some power to influence prices has become common [...]. Facing his weakness in the ability to make contracts, the worker never had doubts about the appropriate solution, which was to organize a union. The vision of the farmer regarding his problem and its solution has never been very defined [...]. Voluntary organizations to expand their economic power - cooperatives - seemed to be the solution at some moments" [11]. For a more complete comprehension of the theoretical perspective of development, see Furtado [12].

[5] After the democratization process, more specifically from the year 1994 (the date of the promulgation of the new antitrust Brazilian law, the Brazilian System of Defense of Competition – SBDC) on, it began to become apparent through analysis of acts of concentration. Many famous trials became paradigmatic examples, as the acts of concentration involving Kolynos and Colgate (AC no. 0027/1995), Antarctica and Brahma - AMBEV (AC no. 08012.005846/99-12) and, more recently, Nestlé and Garoto (AC no. 08012.001697/2002-89). By analyzing acts and contracts that may have an impact on competition, in accordance with the procedure laid down in Article #54, caput and 3rd paragraph of the Law n. 8.884, members of SBDC exert its preventive function, whose objective is to prevent the possible formation of a market power that will enable a possible future abuse perpetrated by the resulting company […]. The members of SBDC also have legal competence to repress anti-competitive behavior, which constitutes its repressive function. In fact, after a start widely focused on analysis of acts of concentration, from 2003 on there was a strong trend towards the actions of public officers in the fight against cartels. This happened especially with the effective use of agreements of leniency, as well as advanced techniques of research, such as the search and seizure and the telephone interception. In order to punish the proven anticompetitive conduct, components of SBDC may impose financial and non-financial penalties" [14].

[6] "According to Kalecki, a normal feature of the economy is operating with idle capacity due to its degree of monopolization. Thus, production takes place not where the price equals the marginal cost, but where it gives the maximum profit. Considering the existence of idle capacity and given the characteristics of the production,

prices, with subsequent restriction of purchases, is inversely proportional to the competition. This rule is well-known, so that the price at which the companies offer their goods and services depends on their direct costs and on the price of its competitors, as in $p = mu + np^*$, in which p is the price, p^* is the price of the goods or substitute service (weighted average of prices of all firms competing within the structure of the market), u stands for direct costs and m for a positive margin (*mark-up*) on these costs. In order, n stands for a coefficient of market power within the range $0 < n < 1$, so that the smaller the size and the market power of the Company, p^* converges more to p and the quantities produced approach more the level that could be achieved were it not for the influence of the monopolization degree [16].

By dividing the formula of mark-up rule by u we obtain the following equation of a straight line, in which m converts the linear coefficient of an affine function (Equation 2) with vertical effect – as indicated in the graphic above.

$$\frac{p}{u} = m + \frac{np^*}{u} \tag{2}$$

Plotting p/u and p^*/u in a coordinated axis, it is possible to observe (Figure 1) that direct costs (u) remain constant when m grows. That is, when the degree of monopoly rises, the straight AB moves upward ($A'B'$), or, if it decreases, it moves down to ($A''B''$). This representation adopts the line of 45° ($0K$) as the axis on which $p/u = p^*/u$ and by which i, I' and I'' are marked. The projection on the abscissa is directly proportional to the degree of monopolization. In the stretches of straight lines AB to the left of the shaft $0K$, the ratio of prices to direct costs of the company is greater than the set of competitors. We did not exhaust the possible inferences from this model when u varies from company to company or according to their market power, or when m is equal to the average degree of industry, turning the company into an industry representative.

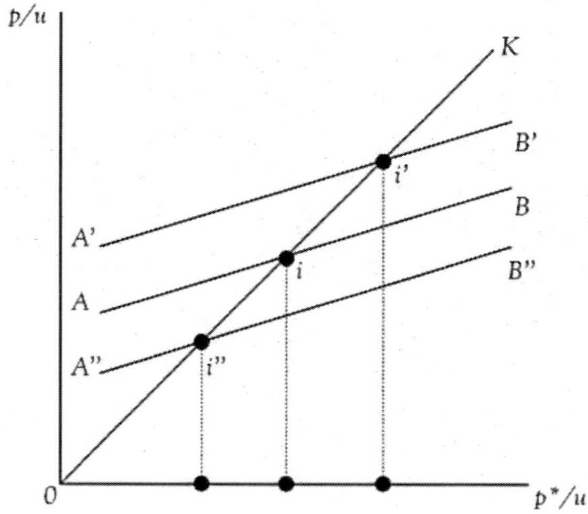

Figure 1. Modification of the Monopoly Degree [16].

there is a horizontal follow-up on the curve of marginal cost, and the price is determined by a margin on costs according to a rule of *mark-up*" [15].

EMPIRICAL INSTRUMENTS

Knowing that the smaller the number of companies and the more unequal the size distribution between them, the less competitive and more concentrated the market is, there are many ways to measure *m* and *n*. Among them is the *Herfindahl-Hirchman Index* (HHI) method, which is used in the United States in one of its variants, of which the usual formula of Hannah and Kay (1977) is the general case (Equation 3). Its index is mathematically given by

$$HK_{NE}(\propto) = (\sum_{i=1}^{n} S_i^{\propto})^{\frac{1}{(1-\propto)}} \tag{3}$$

S_i stands for the market share (the percentage of the market/industry of each of the *i-th* firms), *n* for the number of firms, $0 < \alpha \neq 1$ and the subscribed *NE* indicates that its result is calculated in such a way as to present the response in terms of the *Equivalent Number*. What matters to highlight here is just that *m* and *n* are determinable and are often known, and that they can and should fall, every time the interests of the society are taken into account (offended by speculative shortage and/or goods and services that are artificially made more expensive), given any *market power m* or *n*. Based on these calculations, it is possible to identify an environment likely to host abuses from the industry that demands solid waste in Brazil.

An orientation to the use of Excel for the calculation of this index for any industry can be found in P. Latreille and J. Mackley [17]; their model to the Excel simulation spreadsheet (Figure 1), calculating several measures of industrial concentration, plus concentration and Lorenz curves for user-supplied market share/sales values, is available on *International Review of Economics Education* v. 10, Issue 1, pp. 117-127:

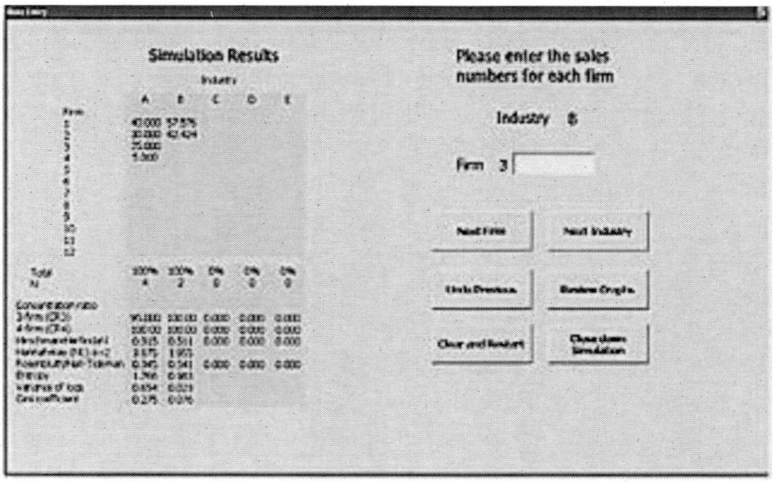

a

Figure 2. (Continued).

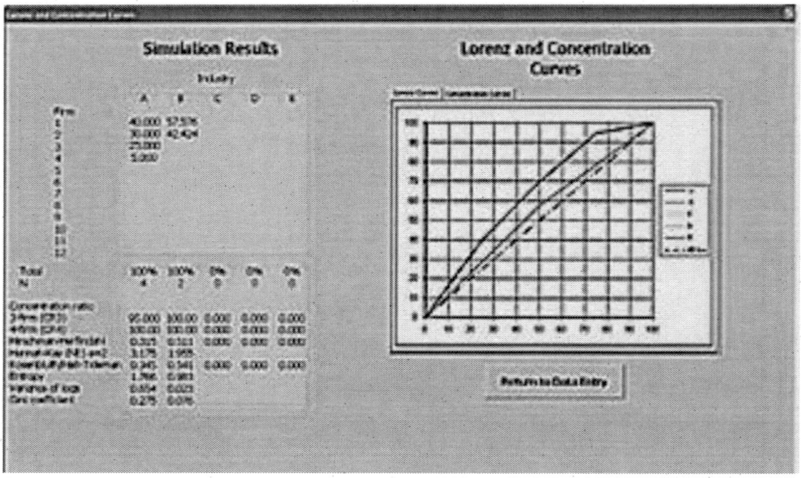

b

Figure 2. (a) The data entry/simulation results screen; (b) Lorenz Curves [17].

The freely available *Excel spreadsheet* allows the user to enter data on market sales by firm for up to 12 firms and up to five industries/markets, which are automatically converted to market shares. Many of the main measures of industrial concentration can be calculated by the program.

Once the data is entered for each of the firms in a particular industry, clicking 'Next Industry' then allows data for the next industry to be entered. For each industry entered, the spreadsheet not only calculates the values of each of the concentration measures listed in Table 1, as noted, but also draws the associated Lorenz curve for each industry/market – the latter being obtained by clicking the 'Review Graphs' button (see Figure 2). This facilitates both statistical and graphical comparisons of the chosen markets. Its *User Guide: Industry Concentration Simulations* gave the following instructions: it is best to download and save this application before you begin. Depending on your settings, the application may not work in your web browser. Before starting the application it is possible that your Excel security settings are set too high to run it, so you should check your macro security settings before opening the file.

Applying similar methods of calculation with Excel spreadsheets, they made it possible to obtain physical and financial results that are significant for the *Complexo Cooperativo de Reciclagem da Bahia* (CCRB), in northeastern Brazil, where the market of solid waste is still highly concentrated by side demand and largely individualized on the supply side [18]. The CCRB acted as a regulator of minimum prices. A solidary credit policy of the *Superintendência de Economia Solidária* provided a re-engineered system of flows and stocks that virtually neutralized the cartel and returned to freelance workers or associates almost any markup of intermediate buyers, with positive externalities for the environment and elimination of exploitation of the poor. The middlemen were no match, then, except through the very short term pricing strategy, to which the CCRB can loosely answer, in one case, raising the price of a kilogram of R$ 1.00 aluminum can for R$ 1.30, increasing almost ten times the physical billing. In most cases, the raise was from R$ 1.30 to R$ 1.50, with no less dramatic results.

CONCLUSION

It is now possible, practical and easy to calculate the degree of industrial concentration in the solid waste market in metropolitan regions of Brazil with Excel.

A second step is the *innovative proposal* to directly connect the networks of cooperatives to the industries. This might happen through contracts, with the stipulation of minimum selling prices (on the part of the associated recyclers) for each residue, which shall be adjusted quarterly by a *tripartite commission joined by representatives of public authorities, civil society and business.* The goal is to define values of products or services according to Article #2 of the Decree n. 7.358. This law redefined fair trade thus:

> I - fair trade: different commercial practice based on the values of social justice and solidarity held by solidary economic enterprises; [...]; V - fair price: is the definition of value of the product or service, built from the dialogue, transparency and effective participation of all the actors involved in its composition that results in equitable distribution of gain in the productive chain. *Only Paragraph* - The terms fair trade, fair exchange, equal fair, alternative trade, solidary trade, ethical and solidary trade are understood inside the concept of fair trade, according to the terms of this Decree [19].

Here we showed a useful instrument against the exercise of power through oligopsony in the reverse logistic of solid waste. We aim to nationally eliminate the *Oligopsonic Exploitation* of recyclers (Trajectory of the Minimum price to *Fair Trade*). This might happen by integrating regional markets through the federal administration of the price of each recyclable element, through the unrestricted and operational use of Excel.

The application of these tools is possible in all highly concentrated markets. The policy maker, however, can only draw regulatory strategies in the face of a specific institutional setting, which is often challenging.

REFERENCES

[1] Furtado, C. (1996). *O Mito do Desenvolvimento Econômico* (The Myth of Economic Development). Rio de Janeiro: Paz e Terra.

[2] Magera, M. (2008). *A Reciclagem dos Resíduos Sólidos Urbanos e o Uso das Cooperativas de Reciclagem: Uma Alternativa aos Problemas do Meio Ambiente* (The Recycling of Solid Waste and Recycling Use of Cooperatives: An Alternative to the Problems of the Environment). Recuperado de http: www.fundace.org.br/cooperativismo/arquivos_pesquisa_ica_la_2008/043-magera.pdf.

[3] Freitas, L., Fonseca, I. (2012). *Diagnóstico sobre Catadores de Resíduos Sólidos: Relatório de Pesquisa* (Diagnosis of Collectors of Solid Waste: Research Report). Brasília: IPEA.

[4] Carmo, M. (2011). As Políticas de Estimulação ao Trabalho dos Catadores no Rio de Janeiro Como Estratégia Oriunda da Valorização dos Resíduos (The stimulation policies to work of Collectors in Rio de Janeiro As Strategy Coming from Waste Recovery), *Cadernos Gestão Pública e Cidadania* (Notebooks Public Management and Citizenship), v. 16, n. 58. São Paulo.

[5] Grimberg, E., Tuszel, L., Goldfarb, Y. (2004). *Gestão Sustentável de Resíduos Sólidos e Inclusão Social:* Estudo de caso sobre as Cooperativas das Centrais de Triagem do Programa Coleta Seletiva Solidária da Cidade de São Paulo (Sustainable Management of Solid Waste and Social Inclusion: Case Study on the Cooperatives of Screening Centers of the Joint Selective Collection Program of the City of São Paulo). São Paulo: ITCP/USP.

[6] Smith, R. (1985). Troca Desigual e Industrialização no Nordeste (Uneven and Industrialization exchange in Northeast). São Paulo: IPE.

[7] Dagnino, R, Dagnino, R. (2010). Políticas para Inclusão Social de Catadores de Materiais Recicláveis (Policies for Social Inclusion of Recyclable Materials), *Revista Pegada* – especial, n. 66, julho/2010.

[8] Carmo, M. (2009). *A Semântica 'Negativa' do Lixo Como Aspecto 'Positivo'*: Um Estudo de Caso Sobre uma Associação de Recicladores na Cidade do Rio de Janeiro, Brasil (Semantics 'Negative' Trash Like Appearance 'Positive': A Case Study About Recyclers Association in the city of Rio de Janeiro, Brazil). Administração Pública e Gestão Social, Viçosa (Public and Social Administration Management, Viçosa), v. 1. n. 2, pp. 21-50, abr./jun.

[9] BOSI, A. (2008). *A Organização Capitalista do Trabalho 'Infor*mal': O caso dos catadores de recicláveis, *en Revista Brasileira de Ciências Sociais* (The Capitalist Labour Organization 'Informal': The case of waste pickers, en Journal of Social Sciences), v. 23, n. 67. junho.

[10] Martins, L., Peres, M. (2006). *Economia Solidária*: A Experiência da Cooperativa do Reciclador Solidário de Piracicaba, en Unimep (Solidarity Economy: The Experience of Solidarity Recycler of the Cooperativa de Piracicaba, en Unimep). *Anais. 4ª Mostra Acadêmica* (Anais. 4th Academic Shows), 24 to 26 of October.

[11] Galbraith, K. (1959). *A Economia e a Arte da Controvérsia* (The Economy and the Art of Controversy). Rio de Janeiro: Fundo de Cultura.

[12] Furtado, C. (1979). *Teoria e Política do Desenvolvimento Econômico* (Theory and Policy of Economic Development). São Paulo: CEN.

[13] Coutinho, M. (1993). *Lições de Economia Política* Clássica (Classical Political Economy lessons). São Paulo: Editora Hucitec.

[14] Ragazzo, C. (2007). *Análise Econômica da Regulação*: O Papel da Advocacia da Concorrência. Berkeley Program in Law and Economics (Economic adjustment Analysis: The Role of Competition Law. Berkeley Program in Law and Economics). UC Berkeley: Latin American and Caribbean Law and Economics Association (ALACDE), *Annual Papers*.

[15] Kalecki, M. (1976). *Teoria da Dinâmica Econômica* (Theory of Economic Dynamics). São Paulo: Abril.

[16] Gremaud, A., Braga, M., Vasconcelos, M., Toneto Jr., R. (2000). A Economia Kaleckiana e o Princípio da Demanda Efetiva (The Kaleckian Economy and the Principle of Effective Demand). In: Lopes, L.; Vasconcelos, M. (Orgs.): *Manual de Macroeconomia*: Nível Básico e Nível Intermediário (Macroeconomics Manual: Basic Level and Intermediate Level). São Paulo: Atlas.

[17] Latreille, P., Mackley, J. (2011). Using Excel to Illustrate Hannah and Kay's Concentration Axioms, *International Review of Economics Education* v. 10, Issue 1, pp. 117-127.

[18] Primo, R. (2011). Política Transversal de Regulação do Mercado Oligopsônico de Resíduos Sólidos nos Carnavais de Salvador de 2007 a 2012 por meio de um Complexo de Economia Solidária (Market Regulation Policy Cross Oligopsônico Solid Waste in the Salvador Carnival from 2007 to 2012 through a Solidarity Economy Complex), *Isegoria - Ação Coletiva em Revista*, UFV - Área Temática: Economia Solidária e Cooperativismo (Isegoria - Collective Action in Review, UFV - Thematic area: Solidarity Economy and Cooperatives), Ano 1, vol. 1, n. 2, set. de 2011/fev.

[19] Brasil. Presidência da República. (2010). Casa Civil (Civil House). *Decreto Nº 7.358*, de 17 de novembro de 2010 (Decree No. 7358 of November 17, 2010). Institui o Sistema Nacional do Comércio Justo e Solidário - SCJS, cria sua Comissão Gestora Nacional, e dá outras providências (Establishing the National System of Fair and Ethical Trade - SCJS creates its National Management Committee, and other measures).

In: Models and Methods for Supporting Decision-Making … ISBN: 978-1-63485-173-2
Editors: Carlos N. Bouza, Flávio L. de Mello et al.

Chapter 2

ESTIMATION OF DERIVATIVES, FROM ECONOMY TO ENVIRONMENT: A STUDY OF THE MANAGEMENT OF EUTROPHICATION OF A FRESH WATER BASIN'S DATA

Sira M. Allende-Alonso[1,*], Dan C. Chen[2], Carlos N. Bouza[1], José M. Sautto-Vallejo[3] and Agustín Santiago-Moreno[3]
[1]Mathematics and Computation Faculty, University of Havana, Cuba
[2]Smith and King College, Calcutta, India
[3]Universidad Autónoma de Guerrero, Guerrero, México

ABSTRACT

The use of derivatives is common in Economic studies. Econometricians have developed alternative procedures to estimate derivatives of conditional expectations. They use non parametric approaches. The management of different environment problems are similar to the financial ones. Hence, we tackle the use of them in the environmental issues associated with the contamination of a basin by Eutrophication. This paper is concerned with a comparissone of the influence of derivatives estimators for studying the contamination due to chlorophyll in a basin. The use of direct and indirect methods is discussed. The conclusions are based on the results of a large simulation study developed using collected data on contamination of a basin. A main result is that Bootstrap performs fairly better than the other procedures based on kernels inclusive under asymptotic considerations.

Keywords: derivatives, non-parametric estimation, kernels, Bootstrap

* Corresponding Author address: Mathematics and Computation Faculty, University of Havana, Cuba, C.P. 10400, Vedado. Email: bouza@matcom.uh.cu.

INTRODUCTION

Social scientists and applied economists often use estimations of the derivatives with parametric specifications of the conditional expectation function, m(x). As derivatives are relatively easily computed, for fitting the regression function, the popularity of parametric estimators has been due to the un-knowledge of other more effective methods. The validity of this approach depends on assumptions on the functional form. Advanced econometricians have developed alternative procedures for estimating derivatives of conditional expectations using nonparametric statistical methods. Unfortunately they have slow rates of convergence. The convergence rates depend on the dimensionality and smoothness of the underlying conditional expectation function. In many economical applications appears that constructing adequate statistics and estimate the Average Derivative (ADE) is an adequate model. See the seminal papers of Stoker [25] and Härdle-Stoker [16] on the semi parametric estimation of average derivatives of regression functions.

From a statistical standpoint, the benefit of this additional averaging is the possibility of using tools for deriving asymptotical normality. The most popularly used models are nonparametric techniques, in These issues, are based on kernel estimators. Average derivatives can be estimated by using kernels. Estimators of this kind were proposed by Härdle and Stoker [16]. Unfortunately, often the theory needs of modifications of the kernel based ADE. There is extensive empirical research studying financial derivatives.

The management of different environment problems are similar to the financial ones. Take for example the management of freshwater. It poses complicated questions as it is needed as a source for drinking and agriculture. The water quality is important as a lack of it affects human health. Eutrophication is becoming a serious water quality problem in fresh water basins. Eutrophication is associated with the toxins produced by some algae. They are potentially dangerous as can poison humans and animals that consume contaminated water and food. The chlorophyll concentration is an important parameter in the evaluation of water quality, nutrition status and organic pollution extent. Hence the management depends heavily in effective monitoring water pollution that is costly and time-consuming, even using remote sensing.

In environmental research of water pollution the derivative analysis of spectra seems to be effective for information detection, see Yang et al.[30]. Nowadays is been applied in analytical chemistry, see Ni [22]. It is well known that the use of spectral derivatives allows the elimination of background signals and resolution of overlapping spectral features which scramble the real information.

The objectives of this study is to compare the influence of derivatives estimators for studying contamination due to chlorophyll in a basin.

Section 2 is devoted to the discussion of the use of direct and indirect methods. Section 3 is devoted to the use of an additive model where the multivariate information is modeled by a sum of univariate models. Section 3 present a large simulation study using collected data on contamination of a basin.

ESTIMATING DERIVATIVES: DIRECT AND INDIRECT APPROACHES

Econometricians have developed alternative procedures to estimate derivatives of conditional expectations which are based on nonparametric methods. However, nonparametric methods can have relatively slow rates of convergence. Furthermore convergence rates depend on the dimensionality and smoothness of the underlying conditional expectation function. In many applications, the objective of the analysis is not to predict the entire derivative curve of a conditional expectation function at each data point. Instead, it is often sufficient to construct statistics to estimate the Average Derivative (AD). Commonly the analysis is based on a regression function described as

$$y_t = m(\vec{X}_t) + \varepsilon_t, t = 1, \dots, T;\ \vec{X} \in \Re^k;$$

$$E(\varepsilon_t) = 0, Cov\left(\varepsilon_t, \varepsilon_j\right) = \begin{cases} \sigma_t^2 \ si\ t = j \\ 0\ otherwise \end{cases}$$

This model fixes that

$$E(Y|\vec{X}) = m(\vec{X}).$$

Take $f(\vec{x})$ as the marginal density function of $\vec{X}$.

$$E(\vec{X}) = \vec{\mu}, V(\vec{X}) = \Sigma$$

The derivative is

$$D\left(m(\vec{X})\right) = \frac{\partial m(\vec{X})}{\partial \vec{X}}$$

Its expectation (average derivative, AD) is given by

$$\delta = \int D\big(m(\vec{x})\big)f(\vec{x})d\vec{x} = E(\Lambda(\vec{x})y) = -\frac{D\big(f(\vec{x})\big)}{f(\vec{x})}$$

δ is a functional.

This problem has elegant and easy solutions within the non-parametric work frame.

Kernel Based Solutions

Take the observations $\{(\vec{X}_1, Y_1), \dots, (\vec{X}_T, Y_T)\}$. An estimator of the density using a kernel function $K_h(\vec{X}_t, \vec{x})$ is described by, see Tsybakov [29]:

$$\hat{f}_h(\vec{x}) = \frac{1}{T\prod_{i=1}^{k} h_i}\sum_{t=1}^{T} K_h(\vec{X}_t, \vec{x}) = \frac{1}{T\prod_{i=1}^{k} h_i}\sum_{t=1}^{T} K_h\left(\frac{x_1 - X_{t1}}{h_1}, \ldots, \frac{x_k - X_{tk}}{h_k}\right)$$

K_h is multivariate kernel definded on k arguments. The bandwidth hj commonly are assumed equal for each component and

$$\prod_{i=1}^{k} h_i = h^d.$$

It is popular using as bandwidth matrix a no-singular one H. Then we have the formula

$$\hat{f}_H(\vec{x}) = \frac{1}{Tdet(H)}\sum_{t=1}^{T} K\left[H^{-1}(\vec{X}_t, \vec{x})\right] = \frac{1}{T}\sum_{t=1}^{T} K_H\left[(\vec{X}_t, \vec{x})\right] = \frac{1}{T}\sum_{t=1}^{T} K_H[H^{-1}(u_t)] = \text{Se}.$$

Some common assumptions are

- $\int K(u)du = \int \hat{f}_h(\vec{x})d\vec{x} = 1.$
- $\hat{f}_H(\vec{x}) = \frac{1}{T}\sum_{t=1}^{T} K_H\left[(\vec{X}_t, \vec{x})\right] \xrightarrow{P} f(\vec{x})$

Consider the development in Taylor Series, where He is the Hessian matrix,

$$f(\vec{x} + \vec{t}) = f(\vec{x}) + \vec{t}^T \nabla_f(\vec{x}) + \frac{1}{2} He_f(\vec{x})\vec{t} + o(\vec{t}^T\vec{t})$$

Then we have that

$$E(\hat{f}_H(\vec{x})) \cong \int K(s)\left\{f(\vec{x}) + \vec{s}^T H^T \nabla_f(\vec{x}) + \frac{1}{2}\vec{s}^T H^T \quad He_f Hs\right\} ds$$

$$V(\hat{f}_H(\vec{x})) \cong \frac{1}{Tdet(H)}\int K^2(s)\{f(\vec{x}) + \vec{s}^T H^T \nabla_f(\vec{x})\}ds \cong \frac{\|K(s)\|_2^2 f(\vec{x})}{Tdet(H)}$$

$$AMISE(H) = \frac{\mu_2^2(K)}{4}\int \quad \left[tr\{H^T He_f(\vec{x})H\}\right]^2 d\vec{x} + \frac{\|K(s)\|_2^2}{Tdet(H)}$$

as

$$E(Y|\vec{X}) = m(\vec{X}) = \int \quad y\hat{f}(y|\vec{x})dy = \int \quad y\frac{\hat{f}(\vec{x},y)}{\hat{f}_{\vec{X}}(\vec{x})}dy.$$

$$\hat{f}_{h,H}(\vec{x}, y) = \frac{1}{T}\sum_{t=1}^{T} K_H[(Y_t - y)]K_H\left[(\vec{X}_t - \vec{x}) \quad \right]$$

One of the more popular estimators is Nadaraya-Watson's

$$\widehat{m_H}(\vec{x}) = \begin{cases} \sum_{t=1}^{T} \frac{y_t K_H\left(\frac{\vec{x}_t - \vec{x}}{h}\right)}{\sum_{t=1}^{T} K_H\left(\frac{\vec{x}_t - \vec{x}}{h}\right)}, \; K_H\left(\frac{\vec{x}_t - \vec{x}}{h}\right) \neq 0 \\ 0, otherwise \end{cases}$$

It is the weighted mean of the observations and

$$V\left(\widehat{m_H}(\vec{x})\middle|\vec{X}_1,\dots,\vec{X}_T\right)=\frac{\|K\|_2^2\sigma^2(\vec{x})}{T det(H) f_{\vec{X}}(\vec{x})}(1+o_P(1));\ \sigma^2(\vec{x})=V\left(Y\middle|\vec{X}\ =\vec{x}\right)$$

The Bias and variance are, asymptotically given by, see Tsybakov [29]:

$$Sesgo(\widehat{m_H}(\vec{x})\left|\vec{X}_1,\dots,\vec{X}_T\right.)\cong\frac{\mu_2(K)\nabla_m(\vec{x})^T H\nabla_f(\vec{x})}{f_{\vec{X}}(\vec{x})}+\mu_2(K)tr(H^T He_m(\vec{x})H$$

$$V(\widehat{m_H}(\vec{x})\left|\vec{X}_1,\dots,\vec{X}_T\right.)\cong\frac{\|K\|_2^2\sigma^2(\vec{x})}{T det(H) f_{\vec{X}}(\vec{x})}$$

Some Kernel Estimators of the Derivatives

Take

$$E\left(m'(\vec{x})=\left(\frac{\partial m}{\partial x_1},\dots,\frac{\partial m}{\partial x_k}\right)\right).$$

It comes from models where the mean response depends on $\vec{X}$ only through a linear combination$\vec{\beta}^T\vec{x}$. Hence the average of the derivative δ is proportional to $\vec{\beta}$ and, as $m'(\vec{x})=g(\vec{x}^T\vec{\beta})$

$$\delta=E\left(m'(\vec{x})=E\left(\frac{dg}{d(\vec{x}^T\vec{\beta})}\right)\right)\vec{\beta}.$$

Therefore δ determines a scaled $\vec{\beta}$.

A popular method for estimating δ is due to Härdle-Stoker [16]. It is denominated of "indirect estimation." The estimator is:

$$\hat{\delta}_{HS}=\frac{1}{T}\sum_{t=1}^T\frac{y_t\widehat{Df_h}(\vec{x}_t)}{\widehat{f_h}(\vec{x}_t)}I\left(\widehat{f_h}(\vec{x}_t)>b_n\right)$$

$\widehat{f_h}(\vec{x}_t)$ is a kernel estimator of a density function and y $\widehat{Df_h}(\vec{x}_t)$ is another kernel estimator but of D. Take the indictor function $I\left(\widehat{f_h}(\vec{x}_t)>b_n\right)$, we have the sequence of threshold values $b_n \rightarrow 0$ and we have the asymptotic result

$$\sqrt{T}(\hat{\delta}_{HS}-\delta)\xrightarrow{Law}N\left(0,V\left(D\left(m(\vec{X})\right)\right)-\varepsilon\Lambda(\vec{x})\right)$$

When the errors do not depend of the regresors

$$V(\hat{\delta}_{HS}) = V\left(D\left(m(\vec{X})\right)\right) + \sigma_{\varepsilon}^{2} E(\Lambda(\vec{x}))^{2}$$

Stoker [25] developed the so called "direct estimator" given by using the plug-in rule

$$\hat{\delta}_S = \sum_{t=1}^{T} \frac{\widehat{D}\left(m(\vec{X})\right)}{T} I\left(\widehat{f}_h(\vec{x}_t) > b_n\right)$$

$\widehat{D}\left(m(\vec{X})\right)$ is a kernel estimator of $D\left(m(\vec{X})\right)$ and

$$\sqrt{T}(\hat{\delta}_S - \delta) \xrightarrow{d} N\left(0, V\left(D\left(m(\vec{X})\right)\right)\right)$$

Both estimators $\hat{\delta}_{HS}$ y $\hat{\delta}_S$ are asymptotically equivalent, see Li [19].

Additive Models

The use of additive models in nonparametric regression analysis is used frequently. Additivity is a way of expressing strong separability which allows to model analysis, interpretation and decision making. Stone [26, 27] derived that additive regression models can be estimated at the univariate rate of convergence. This approach allows escaping from the "curse of dimensionality." It is no longer valid if the impact of the regressors on the response can be considered as separable. The regression function E [Y |X] = m(X) is additive if

$$Y_t = c + m(\vec{X}_t) + \varepsilon_t = c + \sum_{b=1}^{B} f_b \ (X_b)$$

where

$$t = 1, \ldots, T;\ \vec{X} \in \Re^k;$$

$$c \ a \ known \ constant$$

$$f_b \ \ are \ unknown \ functions, b = 1, .., B.$$

Assume that the functions are smooth. If this is not the case, arbitrarily up to the identifiability condition

$$\forall b = 1, \ldots, B, E(f_b \ (X_b)) = 0.$$

There are different procedures. We may mention the back fitting of Hastie and Tibshirani [17]; Mammen et al. [21] and series estimator of Andrews and Whang [1], the marginal integration estimator of TjHstheim and Auestad [28]. The common feature is that they appeal to the dialectical wellbeing of the practical and theoretical sides, because of simplicity in implementation and sound based theory.

In many cases we deal with binary data, the logarithm transform of Poisson count data, etc. Then is used a monotone link function and the techniques associated to the logit and probit links, loglinear, for example. Consider that the link function G (·) is known a priori and we model it as

$$G\big(m(x)\big) = \sum_{b=1}^{B} f_b \ \ (X_b)$$

Now the component functions are univariate. Hence is usable the local polynomial estimation scheme for the components f_b. For inferring on the derivative we must express it in terms f_b^v, of the known G and of the unknown function m. Take

$$F_a \ \ (x_a) = c + f_a(x_a), a = 1, \dots, B$$

then

$$G\big(m(x)\big) = \sum_{b=1}^{B} F_a \ \ (x_a) - (B-1)c$$

Denote the variable X = (X_a; $\bar{X}$) where$\bar{X} = (X_1, \dots, X_{a-1}, X_{a+1}, \dots, X_B)$, then we deal with a particular direction *a*.

Taking derivatives on both sides and working by induction is obtained that, see Yang et al. [30],

$$f_a^{(v)}(x_a) = v! \sum_{(j_1,\dots,j_v)\in J_v} G_a^{\sum_{t=1}^{v} j_t}\big(m(x_a+\bar{x})\big) \prod_{l=1}^{v} (\partial_a^l\, m(x_a+\bar{x}))^{j_l}/(j! \ \ )^{j_l} j_l!$$

where

$$J_v = \{(j_1, \dots, j_v) | \quad 0 \le j_1, \dots, j_v \in J_v \le v;\ j_1 + 2j_2 + \dots + j_v \le v\}$$

is a function of the vector variable and is reduced to a function of a scalar variable x_a., Lemma 1 of Yang et al. [30], and

$$f_a^{(v)}(x_a) = \frac{1}{n} \frac{\sum_{i=1}^{n} G_a^{\sum_{t=1}^{v} j_t}(m(x_a+X_i)) \prod_{l=1}^{v} (\partial_a^l m(x_a+\bar{x}))^{j_l}}{(j! \ \ )^{j_l} j_l!} + O_P\left(\frac{1}{\sqrt{n}}\right)$$

This result allows deriving estimators with low-dimensional rates typical for the dimension of the considered derivative function.

Statistical inference in regression uses a sample (X_i; Y_i), i=1; 2; …, n. Generally it is independent and identically distributed sample of model

$$G\big(m(x)\big) = c + \sum_{b=1}^{B} f_b \ \ (X_b)$$

Let us fix some regularity conditions on the kernel functions:

A1. The kernel K (·) is a symmetric, compactly supported and a Lipschitz continuous probability density; while the kernel L (·) is symmetric, compactly supported and Lipschitz continuous with ∫L (u) du = 1 and order q where q > (B - 1)/4 for estimating and q > (d - 1) ((p + 1) = (p + 3v)) for testing hypotheses
A2. The bandwidths satisfy nh_{gB-1} = ln (n) →∞, g_{2q}/h_{p+1} → 0 and h = $h_{0p\ n-1}$/ (2p + 3) for estimation and h = h_t = h_{0n-2}/(2p + 3v + 2) for testing hypotheses.
A3. The functions f_s (·)'s have bounded Lipschitz continuous (p + 1)th derivatives.
A4. The variance function, $\sigma^2(\cdot)$, is bounded and Lipschitz continuous.
A5. φ y φ* are uniformly bounded away from zero and infinity and have bounded Lipschitz continuous (p + 1)th derivatives.
A6. G is uniformly bounded away from zero and infinity and have bounded Lipschitz continuous (p + 1)th derivative.

Let us take

$$f_a^{(v)}(x_a) = \frac{v!\sum_{i=1}^{n} G_a^{\sum_{t=1}^{v} j_t}(m(x_a+X_i))\prod_{l=1}^{v}(\partial_a^l m(x_a+\bar{x}))^{j_l}}{n\,(j!\ )^{j_l} j_l!}$$

$$f_a\ (x_a) = \widehat{F_a}\ (x_a) - \frac{\sum_{i=1}^{n}\sum_{b=1}^{B}\ \widehat{F_{ib}}(X_b)}{nB}$$

Then the limiting distribution of an adequately centered function of an estimator is a Gaussian. The result is

$$\sqrt{nh^{2v+1}}\left(\hat{f}_a^{(v)}(x_a) - f_a^{(v)}(x_a) - h^{p+1-v} b_{va}(x_a)\right) \rightarrow_{Law} N\left(0, V_{va}(x_a)\right)$$

where

- $b_{va}(x_a) = \frac{v!\mu_{p+1}(K_v^*)}{(p+1)!}\int (G' o\ m)\partial_a^{(p+1)} m(x_a, \bar{x})\bar{\varphi}(\bar{x})d\bar{x}$
- $V_{va}(x_a) = \frac{(v!)^2\|K_v^*\|_2^2}{(p+1)!}\int (G' o\ m)^2\sigma^2(x_a+\bar{x})\bar{\varphi}(\bar{x})^2 d\bar{x}$
- K_v^*an adequate kernel.

Note that the regressors $X_1,\ldots, X_B$ may be clustered into q≤B (non-overlapping) groups. A new problem is determining adequate groups. That is finding the significant interactions between the original, univariate regressors. The usual way is stop after the second-order interaction for having an evaluation of the behavior of the clustering.

Consider that:

- π(x) is a weight function with Lipschitz continuous (p + 1)th derivative
- $\vartheta = (z_{1-\alpha} + z_{1-\beta})\sigma_S^2, z_{1-q} = percentile\ of\ order\ 1-q\ of\ the\ N(0,1)\ q = \alpha, \beta$
- α = pre – specified significance level, β = pre – specified type II error

- $\sigma_S^2 = \int \left(\frac{\left\| K_v^{*(2)} \right\|_2^2}{2} \int (G^{'} o\, m)^2 \sigma^2 (x_a + \bar{x}) \bar{\varphi}(\bar{x})^2 d\bar{x} \right) \bar{\pi}(x_a)^2 d(x_a)$
- $\rho_n = n^{-1} h^{-(2v+\frac{1}{2})}$

Our problem of hypothesis testing is

$$H_0: \int f_a^{(v)}(x_a)^2 \pi(x_a) dx_a = 0 \; vs \; H_n: \frac{1}{v!} \int f_a^{(v)}(x_a)^2 \pi(x_a) dx_a \geq \vartheta \rho_n,$$

A test statistic for our problem is

$$S_n = \frac{1}{v!^2} \int \hat{f}_a^{(v)}(x_a)^2 \pi(x_a) dx_a$$

The decision rule is given by

$$Reject\ H \quad if\ nh^{2v+\frac{1}{2}} S_n \geq h^{\frac{1}{2}} K_v^{*(2)}(0) \left(\int \frac{(G^{'} o\, m)^2}{\varphi} \sigma^2 (x_a + \bar{x}) \bar{\varphi}(\bar{x})^2 d\bar{x} \right) \bar{\pi}(x_a)^2 d(x_a) + z_{1-\alpha} \; \sigma_S$$

For numerical reasons the usual procedure is to look on lower degrees of derivatives, when possible.

There are two standard ways: estimating the usage of asymptotical results of the test or using some resampling method. Yang et al. [30] recommended applying the wild-bootstrap as developed by Liu [20] or Wu (1986) for a better approximation to the distribution S_n under H_0. Interested readers in details may consult Gozalo and Linton [9], Härdle et al. [15], Sperlich et al. [24].

A Simulation Study of the Quality of the Water in a Basin

The study of the quality of the water in basins is of importance in environmental studies of water pollution. A key factor is the concentration of chlorophyll. It is considered as the most important parameter as it allows determining the water quality, the nutrition status as well as the organic pollution extent.

The biologist commonly use the hyper spectral reflectance as it provides information on the water components, including chlorophyll-a. An emerging approach to laboratory spectroscopic analysis is the use of the derivative method. Some researchers pointed that the first-order derivative is able to remove pure water effects and the second-order derivative can remove suspended sediment effects, see, Han [11]. There is evidence on the effectivity of using first-order derivative spectrum in comparison with the traditional band ratio model. For example Duan [7] compared several semi-empirical algorithms and found that the first-order derivative model performed much better than the band ratio and three-band model. The results of Huang [15] supported that the first-order derivative model also was better than the single-band and band ratio model.

We will consider as variables the reflectance at the wavelengths λ_1, λ_2, λ_3 and λ_4 denoted X_1, X_2, X_3, and X_4. We placed

Chlorophyll concentration at measurement t = $Y_t = c + m(\vec{X}_t) + \varepsilon_t = c + \sum_{b=1}^{4} f_b \ (X_b)$

Following the experiments of Cheng et al. [3] in our simulations we generated randomly the λ_j ´s using the existing data and the model tuning method of Zimba and Gitelson [31]. The four-band model was built according to the method of Le [19].

The derivative was computed in a population of 2035 values of its measurement for establishing the contamination of a lake. We used h_1 = (1:0; 1:5; 2:0), h_2 = (1:5; 1:75; 2:0), as in Yang et al. [30] for the kernels determined by

- $K_{NW}(u) = I(|u|) \leq 1,$ Nadaraya-Watson
- $K_E(u) = \frac{3}{4}(1 - u^2)I(|u|) \leq 1,$ Epanechnikov
- $K_G(u) = exp\left(-\frac{u^2}{2}\right)/\sqrt{2\pi},$ Gaussian

See Tsyabakov [29] for a detailed discussion on the properties of these kernels. The hypothesis

$$E\left[\sqrt{nh^{2v+1}}\left(\hat{f}_a^{(v)}(x_a) - f_a^{(v)}(x_a) - h^{p+1-v}b_{va}(x_a)\right)\right] = 0$$

was tested using the limiting distribution and a bootstrap method. In each sample was determined

$$Z_q = \begin{cases} 1 \ if \ the \ hypothesis \ was \ accepted \\ \qquad\qquad 0, otherwise \end{cases}$$

Then was computed

$$\hat{\alpha} = \frac{\sum_{q=1}^{Q} \ Z_q}{Q}$$

The population consisted of 12 035 measurements. Samples of size 100, 300 and 500 were selected and was fixed that Q = 1 000, 2 000, 5 000. In our simulation, we take G to be the standard normal distribution. We compared the procedure of Yang et al. [30] with Härdle-Stoker [16] method.

The simulation model was programmed using the facilities provide by R.

The Table 1 gives important information on the behavior of the methods. The most interesting one is that Bootstrapping is fairly better than considering the asymptotic, inclusive with very large values of Q. The kernel of Epanechnikov has the best behavior in all the combinations of sample sizes and repetitions. The method of Yang et al. [30] is better when the asymptotic normality of the estimators is accepted, while is not to be preferred when

Bootstrapping. Bootstrapping, in any case, is better than assuming that the normality assumption holds.

Table 1. $\widehat{\alpha} = \frac{\sum_{q=1}^{Q} z_q}{Q}, \alpha = 0,05, \beta = 0,25$

	Yang et al.		Härdle-Stoker		Yang et al.		Härdle was fixed Stoker		Yang et al.		Härdle-Stoker	
	Asymp.	Btrap.	Asymp.	Btrap.	Asymp.	Btrap.	Asymp.	Btrap.	Asymp.	Btrap.	Asymp.	Btrap.
Q	1 000				2 000				5 000			
					$K_{NW}(u)$							
100	0,22	0,16	0,27	0,10	0,20	0.14	0,24	0,10	0,18	0.11	0,22	0,10
300	0,20	0,14	0,24	0,10	0.20	0,14	0,17	0,10	0,16	0,10	0,13	0,08
500	0,15	0,08	0,18	0,09	0.12	0,10	0,16	0,06	0,16	0,07	0,13	0,05
					$K_E(u)$							
100	0,17	0,07	0,15	0,11	0,16	0,08	0,11	0,10	0,10	0,08	0,10	0,10
300	0,11	0,07	0,10	0,08	0.14	0,07	0,11	0,08	0,06	0,06	0,10	0,08
500	0,10	0,06	0,10	0,08	0,10	0,05	0,08	0,06	0,06	0,05	0,10	0,08
					$K_G(u)$							
100	0,34	0,21	0,23	0,11	0,22	0,19	0,17	0,10	0,11	0,13	0,12	0,09
300	0,28	0,11	0,23	0,11	0,17	0,15	0.19	0,09	0,11	0,13	0.12	0,09
500	0,14	0,11	0,18	0,10	0,15	0,13	0,16	0,06	0,08	0,10	0,12	0,05

CONCLUSION

We have considered different estimators of the derivatives. The goal of the research was to establish how well these estimators behave, when environmental issues are studied, instead of financial ones. The obtained results sustain that procedures based on the estimation of derivatives seem to perform adequatelly in the enviromental problem studied. From an analysis of the theoretical properties, it was not transparent which estimator exhibited the best performance. A real life problem generated a data set on the quality of the water in a fresh basin. The simulation experiment performed allowed comparing the behavior of the classic asymptotic approximation with the Bootstrap procedure developed in this paper. The estimated coverage of the confidence intervals suggested that the use of Bootstrap provides a better coverage. This fact sustains that the need of using large samples sizes is not so important, as using Bootstrap generated confidence intervals that performs better. The proposal of Härdle and Stoker [16] generally performs better than the procedure of Yang et al. [30] when Bootstrap is used while the contrary is detected with the asymptotic approach.

ACKNOWLEDGMENTS

This research was benefited by the support provided by "P223LH001-029, PROJETO CAPES-MES-CUBA 209/13" and PNCB project "Modelos Matemáticos para el Estudio de Medio Ambiente, Salud y Desarrollo Humano." The authors are grateful of the comments of the referees and editors. They allow improving the initial version of this paper.

REFERENCES

[1] Andrews, D. W. K., and Whang, Y. J. (1990): Additive interactive regression models: circumvention of the curse of dimensionality. Econom. *Theory* 6, 466-479.

[2] Brooks, Robert (2010). *"Advanced Derivatives and Strategies."* Introduction to Derivatives and Risk Management (8th Ed.). Mason, Ohio: Cengage Learning, 483-515.

[3] Chen, C. Q.; Tang, S. L.; Xing, Q. G.; Yang, J. K.; Zhan, H. G.; Shi, H. Y. *A Derivative Spectrum Algorithm for Determination of Chlorophyll: A Concentration in the Pearl River Estuary.* In Proceedings of Geoscience and Remote Sensing Symposium, Barcelona, Spain, 23-28 July 2007.

[4] Cheng, Ch., Y. Wei, X. Sun y Y. Zhou (2013,): Estimation of Chlorophyll-a Concentration in Turbid Lake Using Spectral Smoothing and Derivative Analysis. *Int. J. Environ. Res. Public Health* 10, 2979-2994;

[5] Dette, H., von Liers and Wilkau, C., Sperlich, S., (2001): *A comparison of different nonparametric methods for inference on additive models.* Working Paper 01-28, Carlos III de Madrid, Spain.

[6] Droebesque, J. J., Fine J. (1996): *Inférence non paramétrique.* Les statistiques de rangs. Edition Univ. de Bruxelles, Brussels.

[7] Duan, H. T.; Ma, R. H.; Xu, J. P; Zhang, B. (2010): Comparison of different semi-empirical algorithms to estimate chlorophyll-a concentration in inland lake water. *Environ. Monit. Assess.* 170, 231-244.

[8] Durbin, Michael (2011). *All about Derivatives* (2nd Ed.). New York: McGraw-Hill.

[9] Gozalo, P. L., and Linton, O. B. (2001): Testing additivity in generalized nonparametric regression models. *J. Econom.* 104, 1-48.

[10] Han, L. H.; Rundquist, D. C. (1999): Comparison of NIR/RED ratio and first derivative of reflectance in estimating algal-chlorophyll concentration: A case study in a turbid reservoir. *Remote Sens. Environ.* 62, 253-261.

[11] Han, L. H. (2005): Estimating chlorophyll-a concentration using first-derivative spectra in coastal water. *Int. J. Remote Sens.*, 26, 5235-5244.

[12] Härdle, W., W. Hildebrand and M. Jerison, 1991, Empirical Evidence for the Law of Demand, *Econometrica*, 59, 1525-1550.

[13] Härdle, W., Mammen, E. (1993): Comparing nonparametric versus parametric regression fits. *Ann. Statist.* 21, 1926-1947.

[14] Härdle, W., Marron, J. S. (1991): Bootstrap simultaneous error bars for nonparametric regression. *Ann. Statist.* 19, 778-796.

[15] Härdle, H., Huet, S., Mammen, E., Sperlich, and S. (2001): *Bootstrap inference in semi parametric generalized additive models.* Working Paper 00-70, Carlos III de Madrid, Spain.

[16] Härdle, W. and T. M. Stoker (1989): Investigating Smooth Multiple Regression by the Method of Average Derivatives, *Journal of American Statistical Association*, 84, 408, 986-995.

[17] Hastie, T. J., and Tibshirani, R. J. (1990): *Generalized Additive Models.* Chapman and Hall, London.

[18] Hull, J. C. (2009): *Options, futures, and other derivatives*. Pearson/Prentice Hall, Upper Saddle River:

[19] Le, C. F.; Li, Y. M.; Zha, Y.; Sun, D. Y.; Huang, C. H.; Lu, H. (2009): A four-band semi-analytical model for estimating chlorophyll a in highly turbid lakes: The case of Taihu Lake, China. Remote Sens. *Environ*. 113, 1175-1182.

[20] Liu, R. (1988): Bootstrap procedures under some non i.i.d. models. *Ann. Statist*. 16, 1696-1708.

[21] Mammen, E., Linton, O. B., Nielsen, J. P., (1999): The existence and asymptotic properties of a back fitting projection algorithm under weak conditions. *Ann. Statist*. 27, 1443-1490.

[22] Ni, Y. N. (2004): *Chemometrics in Analytical Chemistry*; Sciences Press: Beijing.

[23] Shi, H. Y.; Xing, Q. G.; Chen, C. Q.; Shi, P.; Tang, S. L. (2007): *Using Second-Derivative Spectrum to Estimate Chlorophyll: A Concentration in Turbid Estuarine Waters*. In Proceedings of SPIE, Wuhan, China, 15-17 November 2007.

[24] Sperlich, S., TjHstheim, D. and Yang, L. (2002): Nonparametric estimation and testing of interaction in additive models. *Econom. Theory* 18, 197-251.

[25] Stoker, T. M., (1991): *Lectures on Semi parametric Econometrics* (CORE Lecture Series), Core Foundation, Louvain-la Neuve.

[26] Stone, C. J. (1985): Additive regression and other nonparametric models. *Ann. Statist*. 13, 689-705.

[27] Stone, C. J. (1986): The dimensionality reduction principle for generalized additive models. *Ann. Statist*. 14, 90-606.

[28] TjHstheim, D. and Auestad, B. H. (1994): Nonparametric identification of nonlinear time series: projections. *J. Amer. Statist. Assoc*. 89, 1398-1409.

[29] Tsybakov, A. B. (2004): *Introduction a l`estimation non-paramétrique*. Mathematiques and Applications 41, Springer, Berlin.

[30] Yang, L., S. Sperlichb and W. Härdle (2003): Derivative estimation and testing in generalized additive models. *Journal of Statistical Planning and Inference* 115, 521-542.

[31] Zimba, P. V.; Gitelson, A. A. (2006): Remote estimation of chlorophyll concentration inhypereutrophic aquatic systems: Model tuning and accuracy optimization. *Aquaculture*, 256, 272-286.

In: Models and Methods for Supporting Decision-Making ... ISBN: 978-1-63485-173-2
Editors: Carlos N. Bouza, Flávio L. de Mello et al.

Chapter 3

MODELING ENVIRONMENTAL PHENOMENA AND MEDICAL CLASSIFICATION OF PATIENTS: CASE STUDIES

Carlos N. Bouza[*]
Departamento de matemática aplicada, Facultad de matemática y computación,
Universidad de la Habana, Cuba

ABSTRACT

The use of quantitative methods for implementing the management of environmental and medical problems is common. However, many environmental and medical applications needs using, sophisticated modeling, for implementing adequate decision procedures. In this chapter we present a study of biodiversity and of patient classification. Both problems use indexes and statistical studies about them are developed. They lead to an evaluation of their behavior. The studies are concerned with the construction of strata, for studying biodiversity issues, and with the classification of patients visiting hospitasl with pneumonia.

Keywords: mathematical modeling, quantitative studies, classification

"Commonly statistical models are used in an attempt of explaining the nature of the phenomena that generated the observations."

INTRODUCTION

Health is determined not only by genes but also by the environment where the persons live. Investigation with patients is complex and the key aims of ecological studies is

[*] Corresponding author: bouza@matcom.uh.cu.

integrating the monitoring and assessment of ecological and environmental indicators with effective management practices.

In qualitative research the aim is obtaining a complete and detailed description. The researchers may only know roughly in advance what they are looking for. The related process is inductive and the researcher derives abstractions, concepts, hypotheses, and theories from details. In quantitative research the aim is classifying features, counting and constructing. The need of explaining the nature of the different phenomena, commonly, statistical models are used for modeling the observation-generating mechnism. Quantitative data is more efficient as the researchers are able to test hypotheses, but they may miss contextual detail while qualitative data is richer, more time consuming, and less able to be generalized. Quantitative research is inclined to be deductive and tries to test the validity of some theory. The use of quantitative methods in medicine has an old and fruitful history. They are based on the use of systematic processes for gathering and statistically analyzing the information that has been measured by an instrument. The instruments are used for deriving numbers from the information. Broadly speaking, quantitative research is considered as objective whereas qualitative research often involves subjectivity.

This contribution tries to give an overview of results obtained in our recent research for solving practical issues. Some ideas of the perspective work are given as well as on the research we are actually coping with.

Following, in this chapter, section 2 presents models for quantifying biodiversity. The use of indexes is developed together with their properties. The third section is concerned with the evaluation of an index for classifying patients of acquired pneumonia. The two studies solved real life problems and open new research for completing the unsolved issues.

ENVIRONMENTAL STUDIES: BIODIVERSITY

Biodiversity is globally recognized as a cornerstone of healthy ecosystems, and biodiversity conservation is increasingly becoming one of the important aims of environmental management. Ecologists must use a quantitative measure for measuring biodiversity. The posed problem was establishing a procedure for dealing with the characterization of the diversity in Sierra de Guerrero, Mexico. In this case the interest was in the diversity of the flora in terms of the species present in the sierra. The existence of many different measures of diversity is confusing. Though the formulae differ they have some common characteristics. In [11] is suggested that there is a need of developing empirical studies for establishing the behavior of the different indexes. See also [8] and [9].

The Simpson index [16] is very popular among the ecologists.

$$\lambda_S = 1 - \sum_{i=1}^{K} \pi_i^2$$

Denoting by n_i the number of individuals of the specie i and the population relative frequence of the i-th specie π_i, an unbiased estimator of the Simpson index and its variance, see Bouza and Schubert [16] are given by

$$\hat{\lambda}_S = 1 - \sum_{i=1}^{K} \frac{n_i(n_i - 1)}{n(n-1)},$$

$$Var\left\{\hat{\lambda}_S\right\} = \frac{2}{n(n-1)}\left[\sum_{i=1}^{K} \pi_i^2 + 2(n-2)\pi_i^3 - (2n-3)\left(\sum_{i=1}^{K} \pi_i^2\right)^2\right]$$

The variance is estimated unbiasedly by

$$\hat{Var}_1\left\{\hat{\lambda}_S\right\} = \frac{2}{n(n-1)^2(n-2)(n-3)}\left[\sum_{i=1}^{K}\left\{2n^2(n^2+n-3)\hat{\pi}_i^3 - \right.\right.$$

$$\left. n(5n^2-3n-3)\hat{\pi}_i^2 + 3n(n-1)\hat{\pi}_i\right\} -$$

$$\left. - n^3(2n-3)\left(\sum_{i=1}^{k} \hat{\pi}_i^2\right)^2 + 2(2n-3)\sum_{i<j} n^2 \hat{\pi}_i^2 \hat{\pi}_j + n^2 \hat{\pi}_i \hat{\pi}_j^2 - n\hat{\pi}_i \hat{\pi}_j\right]$$

$$= \frac{2}{n}\left[\sum \left\{C_1\hat{\pi}_i^3 - C_2\hat{\pi}_i^2 + C_3\hat{\pi}_i\right\} - C_4\left(\sum_{i=1}^{K} \hat{\pi}_2^2\right)^2 + \sum_{i<j} C_5\hat{\pi}_i^2\hat{\pi}_j + C_5\hat{\pi}_i\hat{\pi}_j^2 - C_6\hat{\pi}_i\hat{\pi}_j\right]$$

The estimation of the Simpson index using *m* sites selected independently, see [4] is.

$$\hat{\lambda}_{SS} = \sum_{j=1}^{m} \frac{\hat{\lambda}_j}{m}$$

Taking n_{i+}^* as $n^*_{i+} = \sum_{j=1}^{m} n_{ij}$ $(i = 1,..K)$. This estimator is unbiased and its variance is

$$Var\left\{\hat{\lambda}_{SS}\right\} = \frac{1}{m^2}\sum_{j=1}^{m} Var\left\{\hat{\lambda}_j\right\}, \hat{\lambda}_j = 1 - \sum_{i=1}^{K} \frac{n_{ij}(n_{ij}-1)}{n^*_{.i+}(n^*_{.i+}-1)}$$

where the variance is

$$Var\left\{\hat{\lambda}_j\right\} = \frac{2}{n^*_{+j}(n^*_{+j}-1)}\left[\sum_{i=1}^{K} \pi_i^2 + 2(n^*_{+j}-2)\pi_i^3 - (2n^*_{+j}-3)\left(\sum_{i=1}^{K} \pi_i^2\right)^2\right]$$

Another option is using the combined estimator which is defined as

$$\hat{\lambda}_{SC} = 1 - \sum_{i=1}^{K} \frac{n_{i+}^*(n_{i+}^*-1)}{n^*(n^*-1)}$$

is also unbiased, see [4], and its sampling error is

$$V\left\{\hat{\lambda}_{SC)}\right\} = \frac{2}{n^*(n^*-1)}\sum_{i=1}^{K} \pi_i^2 + 2(n^*-2)\pi_i^3 - (2n^*-3)\left(\sum_{i=1}^{K} \pi_i^2\right)^2$$

The Fager index [9] is defined as $\lambda_F = \frac{N(K+1)-J(K-J)}{2} - \sum_{i=1}^{K} N_i R_i$ where $J \in [0,K)$ is an integer fixed by the ecologist and $R_1,\ldots,R_K$ are ranks. The ranks are assigned to the species in a decreasing order of its importance.

Bouza and Schubert [6] proposed to use the transformation $\lambda^*_F = \frac{N(K+1)-J(K-J)}{2N} - \sum_{i=1}^{K} \pi_i R_i$

for making it more tractable from a statistical point of view. Taking $\lambda_0 = [N(K+1) - J(K-J)]/2N$ an estimator of this transformed index is

$$\hat{\lambda}_F = \lambda_0 - \sum_{i=1}^{K} \frac{n_i}{n} R_i = \lambda_0 - \sum_{i=1}^{K} \hat{\pi}_i R_i$$

which variance is $Var(\hat{\lambda}_F) = \sum_{i=1}^{K} \frac{R_i^2 \pi_i (1-\pi_i)}{n}$.

When an independent random sample of m sites is selected an unbiased estimator of the Fager index is estimated by $\hat{\lambda}_{FS} = \frac{\sum_{j=1}^{m} \hat{\lambda}_{jF}}{m} = \lambda_0 - \frac{\sum_{j=1}^{m}\sum_{i=1}^{K} R_i n_{ij} / n^*_{+j}}{m}$, where $\hat{\lambda}_{jF}$ denotes the estimator of Fager's in the site j and the sampling error is

$$V(\hat{\lambda}_{FS}) = \frac{\sum_{j=1}^{m} \left(\sum_{i=1}^{K} R^2{}_i \pi_i - \left(\sum_{i=1}^{K} R^2{}_i \pi^2{}_i + \sum_{i \neq i'} R_i R_{i'} \pi_i \pi_{i'} \right) \right) / n^*_{+j}}{m^2}$$

Another alternative is to combine the information and to estimate π_i using $\hat{\pi}_i{}^* = \frac{\sum_{j=1}^{m} n_{ij}}{n^*}$, where $n^* = \sum_{j=1}^{m} \sum_{i=1}^{K} n_{ij}$. As $E(n_{ij}) = n^*_{+j}\pi_i$, $I = 1,..,K$, $j = 1,..,m$, an unbiased estimator is

$$\hat{\lambda}_{FC} = \lambda_0 - \frac{\sum_{i=1}^{K} R_i \hat{\pi}_i^*}{m}$$

and $V(\hat{\lambda}_{FC}) = \frac{\sum_{i=1}^{K} R^2{}_i \pi_i - \left(\sum_{i=1}^{K} R^2{}_i \pi^2{}_i + \sum_{i \neq i'} R_i R_{i'} \pi_i \pi_{i'} \right)}{n^*}$ is its variance.

The Shannon index [14] is given by $\lambda_{Sh} = -\sum_{I=1}^{K} \pi_i \ln(\pi_I)$ and is derived from the proposal of measuring the entropy of a system. The Shannon index $\lambda_{Sh} = -\sum_{i=1}^{K} \pi_i \ln(\pi_i)$ is used frequently because its roots are justified, in physics, by its role in measuring entropy. An estimator of it, see Hsieh and Li (1998), is $\hat{\lambda}_{Sh} = -\sum_{i=1}^{K} \hat{\pi}_i \ln(\hat{\pi}_i)$. They studied its behavior when a random sample is selected and established that it is a maximum likelihood estimator. Its variance is given by:

$V(\hat{\lambda}_{Sh}) = \frac{1}{n}\left[\sum_{i=1}^{K}(\pi_i \ln(\pi_i))^2 - \lambda_{Sh}^{\;2}\right]$, if m independent random samples are selected the use of the separate estimator $\hat{\pi}_{ij} = \frac{n_{ij}}{n^*_{+j}}$ yields, as a naïve estimator $\hat{\lambda}_{ShS} = -\sum_{j=1}^{m} \frac{\sum_{i=1}^{K} \hat{\pi}_{ij} \ln(\hat{\pi}_{ij})}{m} = \frac{\sum_{j=1}^{m} \hat{\lambda}_{Shj}}{m}$. Hence if $V_{Shj} = \frac{1}{n^*_{+j}}\left[\sum_{i=1}^{K}(\pi_{ij} \ln(\pi_{ij}))^2 - \lambda_{Shj}^{\;2}\right]$ $j = 1,..,m$ the variance of the estimator is $V(\hat{\lambda}_{ShS}) = \frac{1}{m^2}\left[\sum_{j=1}^{m} V_{Shj}\right]$. Using the combination of the counts of the samples the corresponding combined estimator considered is $\hat{\lambda}_{ShC} = -\frac{\sum_{i=1}^{K} \hat{\pi}_i^* \ln(\hat{\pi}_i^*)}{n^*}$ and its variance can be estimated by $V_{ShC} = \frac{1}{n^*}\left[\sum_{i=1}^{K}(\hat{\pi}_i^* \ln(\hat{\pi}_i^*))^2 - \hat{\lambda}_{ShC}^{\;2}\right]$.

The survey developed in Sierra de Guerrero did not consider the existence of zones with a differentiated diversity. For establishing a monitoring network it is necessary to establish the homogeneity of them. As samples are selected, the clustering of the zones is made after sampling. We look for groups of homogeneous zones. The indexes λ_t, t = 1, 2, 3, are considered as the variables of interest. A stratum (homogeneous zone) is considered as a set of population units such that the evaluation of the biodiversity index, λ_t,(t = 1, 2, 3,) in each sampling unit u_j, is similar. Ideally, once the strata are determined, these parameters must be very different from stratum to stratum. The strata construction is modeled using the results of [2].

The ecologists generally hesitate when considering which index is to going to be used. The determination of strata using the three indexes as stratification variables will produce strata that would satisfy the preferences of them. We considered that in each stratum U_h of size M_h the arithmetic mean if a diversity index t is $\lambda^*t(h)$. The ecologist wants: that for any t:

- $\lambda^*_t(h)$, be close to the individual sample site values.
- $\lambda^*_t(h)$, be very different from the population mean of the index λ^*_t.

The measurement of the number of individuals in a site q provides the vector $\lambda_q = \{\lambda_{q1}, \lambda_{q2}, \lambda_{q3}\}$ while the dispersion of the diversity in the population is measured by $\frac{\sum_{q\in U}(\lambda_{qt}-\lambda_t^*)^2}{M} = \sigma_t^2$ and within the stratum U_h by $\frac{\sum_{q\in U_h}(\lambda_{qt}-\lambda_t^*(h))^2}{M_h} = \sigma_t^2(h)$. The population mean can be expressed by the linear function of the strata means, see [7], $\lambda^*_t = \sum_{h=1}^{H} \gamma_h \lambda_t^*(h)$, $t = 1,..3$, where $\gamma_h = M_h/M = Prob(u_q \in U_h)$, $\forall h = 1,..,H$.

Allende–Bouza [2] proposed the following mathematical programming model for clustering and sampling:

$$P1: Minimize \sum_{q=1}^{M} \sum_{t=1}^{T} \sum_{r=1}^{R} w_t V_{qrt} x_{qr} = \sum_{q=1}^{M} \sum_{r=1}^{R} c_{qr}^* x_{qr}$$

Subject to:

$$\sum_{r=1}^{R} x_{qr} = 1, q \in U;$$
$$\sum_{q=1}^{M} x_{qr} \leq Q_r y_r, r \in R;$$
$$\sum_{r=1}^{R} y_r \leq H,$$
$$x_{qr} \in \{0,1\}, \forall q, r, y_r \in \{0,1\}, \forall r=1,..,R$$

$$x_{qr} = \begin{cases} 1 \; if \; q \; is \; assigned \; to \; U_r \\ 0, otherwise \end{cases}, y_r = \begin{cases} 1 \; if \; \Theta_r \; is \; selected \; centroid \\ 0 \; in \; other \; case \end{cases}$$

where $c^*_{qr} = \sum_{t=1}^{T} w_t V_{qtr}$.

The first constraint establishes that each sample site belongs only to one stratum. The second one fixes that there will not be a stratum with more than Qr units. The third constraint fixes that no more than H strata can be determined. The importance of the t-th variable is weighted by wt. The strata determined by solving P1 may be considered as of minimum multivariate variance because if $\theta_{tr} = \lambda_t^*(r)$, $\frac{\sum_{q \in U_h} V_{qrt}}{M_h} = \sigma_t^2(h)$. Hence the solution of P1 yields an "approximately minimum multivariate variance" stratification. We consider that a sample is selected from U and we determine strata by dividing the sample s into subsamples $s_h = s \cap U_h$ $h = 1 \ldots H$. This technique allows estimating not only λ^*_t but the stratum's parameters $\lambda^*_t(h)$. Our objective is to use the information provided by s to establish a stratification in U. It is basically the idea present in clustering but the difference with the usual post-stratification is that the strata are not known. The optimal stratification procedures in the literature uses T = 1 variables but in our case T>1. As we are using sample information P1 is no longer adequate because we deal with a Stochastic Program.

Albareda et al. [1] suggested a method for determining the deterministic counterpart. The new mathematical program is:

$$P2: Minimize \sum_{q=1}^{M} \sum_{t=1}^{T} \sum_{r=1}^{R} w_t V_{qrt} x_{qr} = \sum_{q=1}^{M} \sum_{r=1}^{R} c_{qr}^* x_{qr}$$

Subject to:

$$\sum_{r=1}^{R} x_{qr} = 1, q \in U;$$
$$\sum_{r=1}^{R} y_r \leq H,$$
$$Prob\left[\sum_{q=1}^{M} p_{qr} x_{qr} \leq b_r y_r\right] \geq 1 - \alpha \; r = 1 \ldots R$$
$$x_{qr} \in \{0,1\} \forall q, r; y_r \in \{0,1\}, \forall r=1,..,R$$

$$x_{qr} = \begin{cases} 1 \; if \; u_q \in s \cap U_r \\ 0 \; in \; other \; case \end{cases}; y_r = \begin{cases} 1 \; if \; \Theta_r \; is \; selected \; centroid \\ 0 \; in \; other \; case \end{cases}$$

Here b_r represents the maximum number of units admissible in U_r and p_{qr} is a Bernoulli random variable with expectation $E'(p_{qr}) = Prob\{u_q \in s \cap U_r\}$. For a fixed *r*, $Prob\{u_q \in s \cap U_r\} = \gamma_r = {}^{M_r}/_{M}$ which is the weight assigned to the *r-th* stratum. The solution of *P*2 determines which strata have high probabilities and a posterior calculus permits to determine the exact value of each stratum *(γ_r)*.

The corresponding Generalized Assignment Problem can be written as:

P3: Minimize $\sum_{q=1}^{M} \sum_{r=1}^{R} p_{qr} c_{qr}^{*} x_{qr}$

Subject to:

$\sum_{r=1}^{R} x_{qr} = 1, q \in U;$
$\sum^{M}{}_{q=1} p_{qr} x_{qr} \leq b_r,, \forall r=1,..,R;$
$x_{qr} \in \{0,1\}, \forall q,r$

where,

$$p_{qr} = \begin{cases} 1 & \text{if } q \in s \cap U_r \\ 0 & \text{otherwise} \end{cases}$$

In this model b_r represents the number maximum of units in U_r and p_{qr} is the needed resource needed by "*q* for performing the job *r.*" As we are using this model for optimal strata construction the parameters and variables have another meaning and

- b_r is an upper bound of the number of units that can be assigned to U_r.
- The first constraint becomes equality for establishing which each unit should be classified in only one stratum.

Note that to assign unit u_i to certain stratum do not depends of t.

We denote $p_{qr} = p_{q\bullet} \; \forall \; q = 1,..,M$. Since $\sum_{q=1}^{M} p_{q\bullet} \leq \sum_{r=1}^{R} b_r$ is valid in our case, *P3* has at least a feasible solution. Haneveld et al. [10] developed a detailed discussion of this problem.

A particular stratum with a set of a distinguished performance of the units may linked with a demand $\sum_{q=1}^{M} p_{q\bullet} x_{qr} = p(r)$ taking this new variable and the effective assignment of the units $M(r) = \sum_{q=1}^{M} x_{\,qr} \; \forall r = 1,..,R.$

Using these results we have a frame for studying the post-stratification problem. Note that we are dealing with information provided by a random sample *s* for determining post-strata. Due to the particularities of the randomness of our data we will use the modification of *P3:*

*P*3: Minimize* $\sum_{q\in s}\sum^{R}_{r=1} c^*_{qr}x_{qr}$
Subject to:

$\sum^{R}_{r=1} x_{qr}=1,\ \forall q\in s$
$Prob\ \{p\,(r)=\sum_{q\in s} p_q\bullet x_{qr}\le b_r\}\ge 1-\alpha,\ \forall r=1,..,R.$
$x_{qr}\in\{0,1\},\ \forall q\in s,\ r=1,\dots,R$

*P*3* is a stochastic problem with probabilistic constraints. Note that $q(r)$ is the sum of independent Bernoulli variables with expectation W_r. Hence it is a Binomial variable with expected value $[p(r)|s]=\sum_{q\in S} x_{qr}\,\gamma_r = m(r)M_r/M$. Using these results we obtain that

$Prob\{\sum_{q\in S} p_q\, x_{qr}\ge b_r\}=\sum_{h=b_r+1}^{m(r)}\binom{m(r)}{h}\gamma_r{}^h\,(1-\gamma_r)^{m(r)-h}$. The DM is able to fix γ_r by determining the proportion of elements expected to be in U_r.

Note that we can determine a quantile of order α using the fact that we are dealing with a Binomial distribution. The usual choice is to calculate $\lambda_r(b_r,\gamma_r,\alpha)=\max\{\beta\in Z|\ Prob\ (\beta)\le\alpha\}$. The r-th constraint is satisfied if $m(r)\le\lambda_r(b_r,\gamma_r,\alpha)$. Hence the deterministic equivalent program of P*3 is:

$$\text{PD1: Minimize}\left\{\sum_{r=1}^{R}\sum_{q\in S} c^*_{qr}\,x_{qr}\,\middle|\ \sum_{r=1}^{R} x_{qr}\ge 1\ q\in S\ \sum_{q\in S} x_{qr}\le\lambda_r(b_r,\gamma_r,\alpha)\ r=1..R\right\}$$

A relaxation of the integer constraints allows to use the classical Transportation Model for solving PD1. The zones determined by the solution permit to establish a network of monitoring sample points. The effect of the management policies is measured by their capability of maintaining a certain level of diversity (calculated by indexes). A level is adequate if it supports the sustainability of forest. Samples will be selected periodically in the network by fixing some sample points in a zone. Because of its homogeneity the number of sampled points will be small. Comparing the results in different moments, it is possible to evaluate the management of the forest in terms of its sustainability.

This model was used in a study in the basin of San Juan river is located at the north of Estado de Guerrero in the Sierra de Guerrero in Mexico. It is has a surface of 33,447 hectares. The 50% of it is covered by vegetation, 25% has no vegetation, 30% is cultivated by farmers and the rest are urbanized areas.

Taking D($v(d)$, P), $d=1,\dots,7$, as the set of indexes of the determined post strata, the corresponding cost for a certain number of post strata P is

$$\varphi(v(d),\,P|z)=\sum^{3}_{t=1}\sum_{r\in D(v(d),P)} m(r)\sum_{q\in U(r)} w_{td}(\lambda_{qrt}-\hat{\lambda}_{trz})^2/m=\sum^{3}_{t=1} V_t.$$

Where, λ_{qrt} is the index λ_t, $t=1,2,3$, evaluated in the site q included in the post strata $U(r)$. $\hat{\lambda}_{trz}$ is the estimate of the same index using the $m(r)$ sites classified in $U(r)$ using the criteria z (z= eparate, **C**ombined); w_{td} is the weight assigned to the index t, $t=1,2,3$, by the vector $v(d)$. The cost of not stratifying is measured by $\varphi(v(d)|z)=\sum^{3}_{t=1}\sum^{M}_{q=1} w_{td}\,(\lambda_q-\hat{\lambda}_{tz})^2/m=\sum^{3}_{t=1} V^*_t$. It is compared with that obtained by using the proposed method. The relative efficiency of the post stratification was measured by using the ratios $\rho\ (v(d),P|z)\cdot =100[1-\varphi(v(d),\ P|z)/\ \varphi(v(d)|z)$.

We have considered $P=5,10,15,20,25,30$ in the study. The results obtained when the separate criteria is used, are given in the Table 1.

Table 1. Relative efficiency of the separate estimators and number of post strata (*NP*) determined

P	ρ(v (1),P|S)	NP	ρ(v (2),P|S)	NP	ρ(v (3),P|S)	NP	ρ(v (4),P|S)	NP	ρ(v (5),P|S)	NP	ρ(v (6),P|S)	NP	ρ(v (7),P|S)	NP
5	10,6	3	12,3	3	14,6	3	15,1	3	25,2	3	28,5	3	10,0	3
10	18,1	7	11,0	3	18,7	5	20,4	6	29,2	6	31,8	6	10,8	6
15	26,8	11	25,5	11	29,6	12	21,5	12	35,9	11	39,4	10	16,3	11
20	26,5	15	32,1	15	39,5	15	22,1	15	39,3	15	41,5	15	21,7	14
25	26,4	15	34,9	15	39,9	15	23,0	15	48,1	15	51,4	15	22,6	19
30	26,8	18	35,2	15	40,1	16	24,6	15	48,2	15	51,5	15	23,0	19

A similar behavior is observed for P when the combines d estimator is used. See Table 2. The use of a larger a weight for the Shannon index is related with smaller gains in accuracy due to the post stratification derived. In both cases the larger gains are given by the use of d = 6 when Simpson index obtains the largest weight and Shannon's is considerably smaller.

Table 2. Relative efficiency of the combined estimators and number of post strata (NP) determined

P	ρ(v (1),P|C)	NP	ρ(v (2),P|C)	NP	ρ(v (3),P|C)	NP	ρ(v (4),P|C)	NP	ρ(v (5),P|C)	NP	ρ(v (6),P|C)	NP	ρ(v (7),P|C)	NP
5	16,3	3	17,4	3	10,2	2	13,6	3	24,0	3	33,4	3	7,0	2
10	16,2	7	19,6	5	18,3	7	19,2	7	35,2	5	36,2	8	7,2	7
15	25,9	13	29,2	12	23,2	10	26,4	13	41,4	9	45,8	8	7,8	12
20	25,9	15	33,9	15	24,2	15	34,5	15	41,6	15	48.3	15	11,0	18
25	26,1	15	33,9	15	24,3	15	34,9	15	41,5	15	48,5	15	15,2	21
30	26,9	22	34,1	16	24,6	20	35,1	15	41,8	12	49,3	15	15,2	24

The analysis of the results suggested to the ecologists accepting the use of the post strata defined by the Combined estimator for $p=20$ and $d=5$.

We consider that it is needed to determine which are the optimal weight, and establishing whether the stratification, derived by using different weight or estimators, may be considered as similar. We are coping with this problem. The line is considering the similarity among the strata determined by a different procedures.

A Medical Study of Disease Management

The Problem

Pneumonia acquired in the community is considered as a grave problem due to the increase of its prevalence. Persons acquire the disease and go to the hospital. The physicians must manage to classify accurately the needs of the patient; the effect of a deficient classification is evident. A patient goes to the hospital and he/she obtains medications and is sent back home. Some of them returns in sever gravity state due to an incorrect diagnosis. A question is if using a simple clinic evaluation allows giving an adequate prognosis of the gravity of the pneumonia of the patient. Having an adequate objective model for the prognosis the severity of the illness would be a good help for dealing with patients acceding to emergency consults of a hospital.

The control variables must be of easy measuring. Was decided using clinic measures. An index was proposed by physicians of the Hospital General Docente Iván Portuondo de San Antonio de los Baños, province of Artemisa, Cuba, see [8].

Internationally are used methods for providing a fast classification of the patients acceding to the consult. The Pneumonia Severity Index (PSI) and CRB-65 are scores used to predict mortality in patients with community-acquired pneumonia (CAP), see [3]. It is unknown how well either score predicts time to clinical stability in hospitalized patients with CAP. Thus, it is also not known which score predicts better the time to clinical stability. They use clinic parameters. The objective of the research was to validate the index proposed by the Cuban physicians. They proposed, on the basis of the international practice and the real possibilities of Cuban hospital using the information provided by a vector $Y_i = (Y_{i1}, \ldots, Y_{i8})$, where:

$$Y_{i1} = \begin{cases} 1 \text{ if mental confusion} \\ 0 \text{ otherwise} \end{cases},$$

$$Y_{i2} = \begin{cases} 1 \text{ if respiration is abnormal} \\ 0 \text{ otherwise} \end{cases},$$

$$Y_{i3} = \begin{cases} 1 \text{ if blood pressure abnormal} \\ 0 \text{ otherwise} \end{cases},$$

$$Y_{i4} = \begin{cases} 1 \text{ if age} \geq 65 \\ 0 \text{ otherwise} \end{cases},$$

$$Y_{i5} = \begin{cases} 1 \text{ if co-morbidity} \\ 0 \text{ otherwise} \end{cases},$$

$$Y_{i6} = \begin{cases} 1 \text{ if there are complications} \\ 0 \text{ otherwise} \end{cases},$$

$$Y_{i7} = \begin{cases} 1 \text{ if providing medicament orally is not possible} \\ 0 \text{ otherwise} \end{cases},$$

$$Y_{i8} = \begin{cases} 1 \text{ if saturation of oxygen} \\ 0 \text{ otherwise} \end{cases},$$

The index used in practice is modeled by

$$I_i = \sum_{j=1}^{8} Y_{ij} = \text{Score of Ariguanabo for patient i}$$

Table 3. Classification of the patients using the score of Ariguanabo

Risk group o	Value of the score	Decision
1	1-2	Treatment at home
2	3-6	Ingress in a room
3	7-10	Ingress in Intensive Care Unit (ICU)

The groups of risk are 3 and a value of the index determines where a patient should be classified. Table 3 allows implementing a decision rule.

In the study the use of the prognosis different factors are present when testing the state of the patient. For each patient were measured:

- Radiologic pattern
- Glycemic measurement at days 1, 3 and 7,
- Permanence in the hospital.

Logistic Regression

The Hospital Iván Portuondo provided a sample of 123 adults patients diagnosed with pneumonia between 2013 to 2014. Of course patients send back home have neither measures of sugar in blood in days 3 and 7 nor permanence in the hospital. Is usual considering that the probability of a "success" is modeled by

$$P_i = E(Y_i=1 \mid X_i) = \frac{1}{1+e^{-(\beta_1+\beta_2 Xi)}} = \frac{1}{1+e^{-Zi}} = \frac{e^{Zi}}{1+e^{Zi}}$$

That is

$$E(Y_i|X_i) = \begin{cases} P_i = \dfrac{e^{Z_i}}{1+e^{Z_i}}, if\ X = 1 \\ Q_i = \dfrac{1}{1+e^{Z_i}}, if\ X = 0 \end{cases}$$

The usual application in medicine comes from the definition of the odds ratio

$$ODDS\ Ratio = \frac{P_i}{Q_i} = \frac{\frac{e^{Z_i}}{1+e^{Z_i}}}{\frac{1}{1+e^{Z_i}}} = e^{Z_i}$$

The slope is used for evaluating the effect of the changes in the odds as a response in the marginal changes in X, (B2 = ΔL/ΔX). The sign determines the direction of the changes. The probability is estimated using its maximum likelihood estimator,

$$\hat{P}_i = \frac{\text{Number of observations if } Y_i = 1 \text{ for a given certain value } X_i}{\text{Total observations with value } X_i} = \frac{n_i}{N_i}$$

The results of the analysis of OR are given in the next tables

An improvement over this baseline is valid in all the cases. As result it is sustained that using model based inferences is more effective than using a null model. The odds for Complete Restitution had high odds in the case of pneumonic splits (almost 7 times more) and interstitial (close to 2) while for Ingress in ICU the higher odds are for Bronco-pneumonia (around 3 times) and for pneumonic splits is almost the same ratio (close to 1).

Table 4. Analysis of OR for Complete Restitution

	Complete Restitution			
	Bronco-pneumonia	**interstitial**	**pneumonic**	**pneumonic+ splits**
OR	0,575	1,982	0,759	6,888
Confidence interval α=0,05%	0,197-1,670	0,705- 5,567	0,329- 1,752	0,601-78,909
	Ingress in ICU			
OR	2,720	0,647	0,567	1,038
Confidence interval α=0,05%	1,162-6,363	0,217- 1,928	0,264- 1,216	0,091-11,803

Table 5. Analysis of OR for Complete Restitution

Response variable complete restitution					
Variable	**coefficient**	***p*-value**	**OR**	**Confidence interval α=0,05%**	
Glycemic 1	0,0541	0,420	1,06	0,93	1,20
Glycemic 3	0,1200	0,094	1,13	0,98	1,30
Glycemic 7	0,0778	0,402	1,08	0,90	1,30
Days of stay	0,2643	0,001	1,30	1,11	1,53
age	0,0121	0,441	1,01	0,98	1,04
FR≤24	-0,2196	0,613	0,80	0,34	1,88
PAS≥90	-0,6682	0,167	0,51	0,20	1,32
Co-morbidity	1,3523	0,037	3,87	1,08	13,81
providing medicament orally	-0,1629	0,725	0,85	0,34	2,11
complications	1,4469	0,007	4,25	1,50	12,08
Age ≥65	0,4414	0,420	1,55	0,53	4,54
SAT O2	-0,3823	0,456	0,68	0,25	1,87
Mental status	-0,2980	0,501	0,74	0,31	1,77

Additional results were derived. The Table 5 fixes some ideas on complete restitution. It is significantly described by a logistic model when are considered, separately, days of stay co-morbidity and complications (which is not informative for decision making). These variables need of a complete evaluation and is not obtainable from a clinic analysis at the classification consult.

When the restitution was analyzed the results are given in the Table 5. It presents the analysis of the fitted logistic regressions. Only the model using complications, days of stay and co-morbidity were significant for describing the restitution. The rest, though important for physicians do not play a role for management. The OR of them and age were the largest. Hence the prediction of their effect is important for management.

The results are given in the Table 6 when the ingress is considered. For the ingress for therapy were significant only providing medicines orally and the saturation of oxygen. The possibility that the patient obtains the medicines orally is largely the most important factor, its

OR is 12 times larger. The saturation has a very large OR. Hence these two factors, measurable at the consult, provide the more important information for managing the ingress.

Taking the variables used in score of Ariguanabo plus glycemic 1 and radiologic pattern we should fit the multivariate logistic model.

$$P\ (Y = 1|\vec{X}_i) = \frac{e^{B_1 + B_2 X_{i1} + \cdots + B_k X_{ik}}}{1 + e^{B_1 + B_2 X_{i1} + \cdots + B_k X_{ik}}}$$

Table 6. Analysis of OR for Response at ingress in ICU

Response at ingress in ICU					
Variables	**coefficient**	**p-value**	**OR**	**Confidence interval α=0,05%**	
Glycemic 1	0,0684	0,271	1,07	0,95	1,21
Glycemic 3	-	-	-	-	-
Glycemic 7	-	-	-	-	-
days of stay	-	-	-	-	-
age	-0,0082	0,541	0,99	0,97	1,02
FR<=24	-0,1636	0,679	0,85	0,39	1,84
PAS>=90	0,0026	0,995	1,00	0,45	2,21
Co-morbidity	0,0787	0,858	1,08	0,46	2,27
providing medicament orally	2,5289	0,001	12,54	2,83	55,54
complications	0,3281	0,534	1,39	0,49	3,90
Age ≥65	0,2388	0,612	1,27	0,50	3,20
SAT O2	1,3943	0,001	4,03	1,73	9,41
Glycemic 1	0,4690	0,230	1,60	0,74	3,44

Table 7. Logit Regression Analysis of Complete Restitution

	Response: complete restitution				
Best model	**variables**	**Coefficient of regression**	**OR**	**P-valor**	**Confidence interval α=0,05%**
Without glycemic 1	Co-morbidity	2,139	8,50	0,005	1,90-37,93
	complications	2,490	12,06	0,001	2,86-50,84
With glycemic1	Co-morbidity	2,114	8,29	0,006	1,85-37,07
	complications	2,463	11,74	0,001	2,76-49,89
Forward Regression	Co-morbidity	1,817	6,15	0,009	1,57-24,17
	complications	2,169	8,75	0,001	2,39-32,08
Descendent Regression	Co-morbidity	1,817	6,15	0,009	1,57-24,17
	complications	2,169	8,75	0,001	2,39-32,08

We analyze the goodness of fit of the different models. See in the Table 7 the results. For complete restitution. An interesting result is that using the measurement of glycemic is unimportant. The variables of significance are co-morbidity and complications. This result contradicts the state of mind of physicians who consider that glycemic provides important information for managing the restitution. For Ingress ICU are of interest not only glycemic 1 but providing medicament orally and saturation of oxygen. Again the information on glycemic may be dropped without affecting the potentialities of the adjusted model. In any case a model where glycemic at the consult is included provides also a good description of the expected success in complete restitution. The techniques for model selection included it.

ROC Curves

Receiver Operating Characteristic (ROC) curve analysis is being used in medicine for more than 5 decades. The ROC curve depicts the quality of a diagnostic marker into two disjoint classes. It illustrates the trade-off between sensitivity and specificity. The Area Under the ROC Curve (AUC) is the most widely used index for the quantification of the performance of a diagnostic marker in the two-class setting. A useful diagnostic marker will result in an ROC curve with AUC close to 1. We use this technique for validating the behavior of our markers. The obtained graphs are the following, Figure 1 and 2.

Table 8. Logit Regression Analysis for Response at ingress in ICU

Best model	**Response: Ingress ICU**				
	variables	**Coefficient of regression**	**OR**	**p-value**	**IC 95%**
Without glycemic 1	providing medicament orally	2,853	17,34	0,001	3,38-89,02
	SAT O2	2,102	8,19	0,002	2,12-31,65
With glycemic 1	providing medicament orally	2,847	17,24	0,001	3,35-88,63
	SAT O2	2,100	8,17	0,002	2,11-31,64
Forward Regression	providing medicament orally	2,413	11,17	0,002	2,44-51,12
	SAT O2	1,925	6,85	0,001	2,16-21,75
Descendent Regression	providing medicament orally	2,413	11,17	0,002	2,44-51,12
	SAT O2	1,925	6,85	0,001	2,16-21,75

The qualitative evaluation of the AUC is

$$\text{Calification of the effectiveness of } AUC = \begin{cases} \text{if} > 0.9 \text{ excellent} \\ \text{if belonging to }]0.8, 0.9] \text{ equally good} \\ \text{if belonging to }]0.6, 0.8] \text{ acceptable} \\ \text{if belonging to }]0.5, 0.6] \text{ deficient} \\ \text{if belonging to } \leq 0.5 \text{ bad} \end{cases}$$

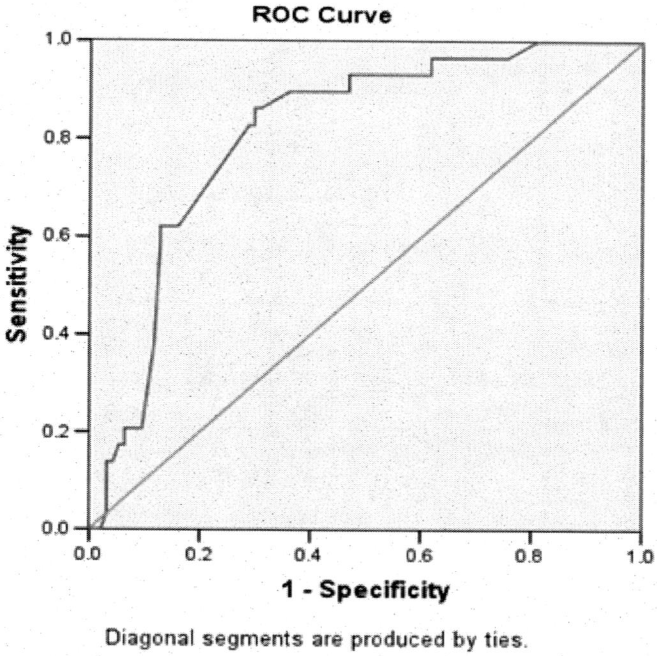

Figure 1. ROC-curve with the response Variable complete restitution and explicative variables of the score of Ariguanabo using the best model. Test Variable predicted probability.

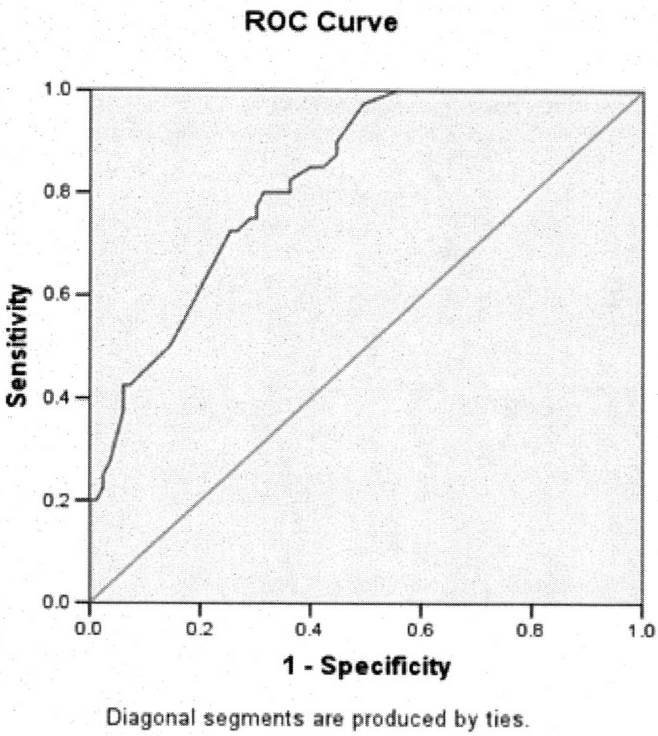

Figure 2. ROC-curve with the response Variable Ingress in ICU and Explicative variables of the score of Ariguanabo using the best model. Test Variable predicted probability.

The description for ingress in ICU fixes that the index is “equally good” as AUC = 0,827 and it was considered as significant. See the Table 9.

The description for complete restitution is considered as “equally good,” as AUC = 0.811, see Table 10.

Table 9. AUC of the response variable “ingress in ICU”

Area Under the Curve

Test Result Variable(s): Predicted probability

Area	Std. Error[a]	Asymptotic Sig.[b]	Asymptotic 95% Confidence Interval	
			Lower Bound	Upper Bound
.827	.036	.000	.755	.898

The test result variable(s): Predicted probability has at least one tie between the positive actual state group and the negative actual state group. Statistics may be biased.

a. Under the nonparametric assumption

b. Null hypothesis: true area = 0.5

Table 10. AUC of the response variable “complete restitution”

Area Under the Curve

Test Result Variable(s): Predicted probability

Area	Std. Error[a]	Asymptotic Sig.[b]	Asymptotic 95% Confidence Interval	
			Lower Bound	Upper Bound
.811	.042	.000	.728	.894

The test result variable(s): Predicted probability has at least one tie between the positive actual state group and the negative actual state group. Statistics may be biased.

a. Under the nonparametric assumption

b. Null hypothesis: true area = 0.5

Table 11. Results derived from the analysis of the ROC´s for the 8 logistic regression equations

	Response: Restitution			**Response: Ingress In ICU**		
Method	**Area ROC**	***p*-Value**	**Confidence Interval $\alpha = 0.05$**	**Area ROC**	**P-Value**	**Confidence Interval $\alpha = 0.05$**
Without Glycemic 1	0.811	0.000	0.728-0.894	0.827	0.000	0.755-0.898
With Glycemic 1	0.813	0.000	0.734-0.892	0.826	0.000	0.755-0.897
Forward Regression	0.785	0.000	0.706-0.865	0.777	0.000	0.696-0.858
Descendent Regression	0.785	0.000	0.706-0.865	0.777	0.000	0.696-0.858

Table 12. Percent of coincidences between the observations and the prognostics. Threshold 0.5

Method	Response: Restitution				Response: Ingress ICU			
		Prognosticated				Prognosticated		
	Observed	0	1	% Correct	Observed	0	1	% Correct
Best Model Without Glycemic 1	0	90	4	95.7	0	71	12	85.5
	1	25	4	13.8	1	20	20	50.0
% Total				76.4				74.0
Best Model With Glycemic 1	0	91	3	96.8	0	70	13	84.3
	1	25	4	13.8	1	20	20	50.0
% Total				77.2				73.2
Forward Regression	0	91	3	96.8	0	71	12	85.5
	1	27	2	6.9	1	24	16	40.0
% Total				75.6				70.7
Descendent Regression	0	91	3	96.8	0	71	12	85.5
	1	27	2	6.9	1	24	16	40.0
% Total				75.6				70.7

Analyzing the Table 11 we have that the same result holds for ingress as AUC = 0.827. Considering if $p > .05$ the null hypothesis that a good model fits to data was tenable for the 8 models fitted. Note that the elimination of variables leads to degrading the qualification of the marker as the AUC becomes only acceptable.

The usefulness of the classification of cases using these models established that the percent correct classification was higher than 75% in the total for complete restitution and for the complete model for ingress in ICU. The cases in which the response Y = 0 was predicted with a very high level of accurateness.

Conclusion

The result of this research allowed evaluating as effective the use of the score of Ariguanabo but poses critics for assigning the same weight to the evaluation of the patient. This study established that the importance of them is very different. This fact should generate further studies for looking for an optimal weighting system.

Acknowledgments

The author acknowledges that he was benefited by the support of the PNCB project Modelos Matemáticos para el Estudio de Medio Ambiente, Salud y Desarrollo Humano and project 209/13 MÊS-CUBA. The comments of referees and editors are acknowledged.

References

[1] Albareda-Sambola, E. and E. Fernández (2000): The stochastic generalized assignment problem with Bernoulli demands. *TOP*, 8, 165-190.

[2] Allende, S.M. and C. Bouza (1987): Optimization criteria for multivariate strata construction, In "Approximation en Optimization" (*Lecture Notes in Mathematics* 1353), 227-233. Springer and N. York.

[3] Arnold F.W., G. N. Brock, P. Peyrani, E. L. Rodrıguez, A. A. Dıaz, P. Rossi, J. A. Ramirez (2010): Predictive accuracy of the pneumonia severity index vs CRB-65 for time to clinical stability: Results from the Community-Acquired Pneumonia Organization (CAPO) International Cohort Study. *Respiratory Medicine* 104, 1736-1743.

[4] Bouza Herrera, C.N. and Covarrubias (2005): Estimación del índice de diversidad de Simpson en m sitios de muestreo. *Investigación Operacional*, 26, 187-195.

[5] Bouza Herrera, C.N., J. F. Garcia, A. Garcia, C. Herrera, T. La Rosa Chibas and P. A. Valdés (2012): Similitud de marcadores predictivos del daño cerebral en hipertensos asintomáticos. *Modelación matemática de fenómenos del medio ambiente y la salud* Tomo 2, 21-32.

[6] Bouza C. N. and Schubert L. (2003): The Estimation of the Biodiversity and the Characterization of the Dynamics: An Application to the Study of a Pest. *Revista de Matematica e Estatistica*. 21, 85-98.

[7] Cochran (1981): *Técnicas de Muestreo*. CECSA, Mexico.

[8] De las Mercedes Larrondo Muguercia H; Jiménez Paneque R; et, al, (2010): Valoración de la glucemia sérica como marcador pronóstico en el paciente séptico crítico, *Revista Cubana de Endocrinología*, 21, 269-278.

[9] Fager, E.W. (1972): Diversity: a sampling study. *American Naturalist*. 106, 293-310.

[10] Klein Haneveld, W. K and M. H. van der Vlerk (1999): Stochastic integer programming: General models and algorithms. *Annals of Operations Research* 85, 39-57.

[11] Kempton, R.A. (2002): "Species diversity," *Encyclopedia of Environmetrics*, 4, 2086-2092. (eds Abbel H. El-Shaarawi and W. Piegorsh) John Wiley and Sons. N. York.

[12] Laurila-Pant M., A. Lehikoinen, L. Uusitalo and R. Venesjärvi (2015): How to value biodiversity in environmental management? *Ecological Indicators* 55, 1–11.

[13] Lim W.S., Van Der Eerden M. and Laing R. (2003) Defining community-acquired pneumonia severity on presentation to hospital: an international derivation and validation study, *Thorax*; 58: 377–382.

[14] Shannon C. E. (1948): A mathematical theory of communication the diversity on. *The Bell System Technical Journal*. 27, 379-423.

[15] Shiver, B. d. and Borders, B. E. (2003): Sampling Techniques for Forest Resource Inventory. J. Wiley, N. York.

[16] Simpson E. H. (1949): Measuring of diversity. *Nature*. Vol 163, 688, doi:10.1038/163688a0.

In: Models and Methods for Supporting Decision-Making ... ISBN: 978-1-63485-173-2
Editors: Carlos N. Bouza, Flávio L. de Mello et al.

Chapter 4

ANALYSIS OF EFFECT OF ENVIRONMENTAL DISCHARGE AND AWARENESS PROGRAMS ON JAPANESE ENCEPHALITIS SPREAD USING MATHEMATICAL MODELING AND SIMULATION

Nita H. Shah[1,*], Urmila Chaudhari[2], Jyoti Gupta[1] and Bijal Yeolekar[1]

[1]Department of Mathematics, Gujarat University, Ahmedabad, Gujarat, India
[2]Department of Applied Sciences, Faculty of Engineering and Technology, Parul University, Vadodara, Gujarat, India

ABSTRACT

In this chapter, the transmission of Japanese Encephalitis (JE) is studied through the system of non-linear differential equation. The effect of environment discharge and awareness program is incorporated to study the spread of the infectious disease. It is assumed that JE spreads when one comes in contact with susceptible and infected mosquitoes only. The awareness program is proportional to the number of infectious. It is assumed that due to awareness programs, susceptible individual form a separate class and avoid contact with infectious. The stability analysis is worked out. Numerical simulation in each compartment is carried out to investigate the spread of the disease.

Keywords: non-linear SEIR-model, Japanese Encephalitis, environment discharge, awareness program, stability analysis

* Corresponding Author address: Email: nitahshah@gmail.com.

INTRODUCTION

Japanese Encephalitis is a viral disease that infects animal and human. It spreads by mosquito bite and results in inflammation of the membrane around the brain. The symptoms are high fever, headache, neck stiffness, coma, seizures and spastic paralysis and ultimate death. JE spreads by the bite of an infected mosquito that has previously sucked blood from an infected animal and person [1]. The risk of transmission is higher in rural areas where pig population is dense and where rice paddles, marshes and standing pools of water supports breeding grounds for mosquitoes and feed for birds. Mukhopadhyay et al. [2] developed a regression equation model using a third order harmonic Fourier series having a linear trend to simulate the spread pattern. Tapaswi et al. [3] modeled the spread of JE in human population of variable size from reservoir population. The reservoir population was considered to be deterministic. It was established that if a threshold exceeds then there exists a unique equilibrium for the disease and gets locally stable if small perturbations occur. The global stability depends on death rates and rates of the equilibrium population sizes of the infected and total human populations. Naresh and Pandey [4] incorporated environmental effects to study the spread of Japanese Encephalitis.

In this chapter, we study the dynamics of Japanese Encephalitis in system consists of human, reservoir and media. It is assumed that the awareness about the disease through media will alert susceptible.

MATHEMATICAL MODEL

These figures must be supplied as separate. The model is developed using following notations for human population, mosquito population, reservoir population and environment/media.

Table 1. List of Variables and parameters

Human Population	
$S_{hu}(t)$	Number of susceptible humans who are unaware at any time t
$S_{ha}(t)$	Number of susceptible humans who are aware at any time t
$E_h(t)$	Number of exposed humans at any time t
$I_h(t)$	Number of infectious humans at any time t
$R_h(t)$	Number of recovered humans at any time t
B_h	Recruitment rate of humans in susceptible class
μ_h	Natural death rate
δ_h	Disease induced death rate
β_h	Probability of transmission of infection from mosquito to human

Human Population	
σ_{huv}	Mosquitoes biting rate to Unaware humans
σ_{hav}	Mosquitoes biting rate to aware humans
ν	Rate of progression of human from exposed class to infectious class
γ	Recovered Rate
α	Rate with which humans become aware
$N_h(t)$	Total human population at any time t
Mosquito Population	
$S_v(t)$	Number of susceptible mosquitoes at any time t
$I_v(t)$	Number of infectious mosquitoes at any time t
B_v	Mosquito's natural growth rate
$N_v(t)$	Total mosquitoes population at any time t
λ_v	Mosquito growth rate due to environmental discharges
μ_v	Natural Death rate
δ_v	Death due to control measure
β_v	Probability of transmission of infection from human/Reservoir to mosquito
Reservoir Population	
$N_p(t)$	Total reservoir population at any time t
$S_p(t)$	Number of susceptible reservoir at any time t
$I_p(t)$	Number of infectious reservoir at any time t
β_p	Probability of transmission of infection from mosquito to reservoir
B_p	Natural recruitment rate of reservoir
λ_p	Reservoir population growth rate due to environmental discharges
μ_p	Natural death rate of reservoir population
δ_p	Death due to control measures
σ_{pv}	Mosquito biting rate of reservoir population
Environment/Media	
W	Conducive environmental discharges
M	The cumulative density of awareness programs driven by media in a particular region
ψ	Rate with which awareness program being implemented
ϕ	Interruption in these programs due to social programs, etc.
B_e	Constant influx of discharges
ω	Rate of growth of environmental discharge due to human activities
θ	Rate of removing/cleaning environmental discharge

Consider the total human population, at any time with birth rate. It is divided into two classes of susceptible viz., non-aware and aware. Both moves to the exposed class and then gets infectious and get a membership of infectious class. The transform diagram for human is shown in Figure 1. The disease spreads due to environment discharge and contact between susceptible human and infectious mosquito. The conductive environment discharge is partitioned to; number of susceptible mosquito and number of susceptible reservoir. Both lead to infectious class as shown in Figure 1.

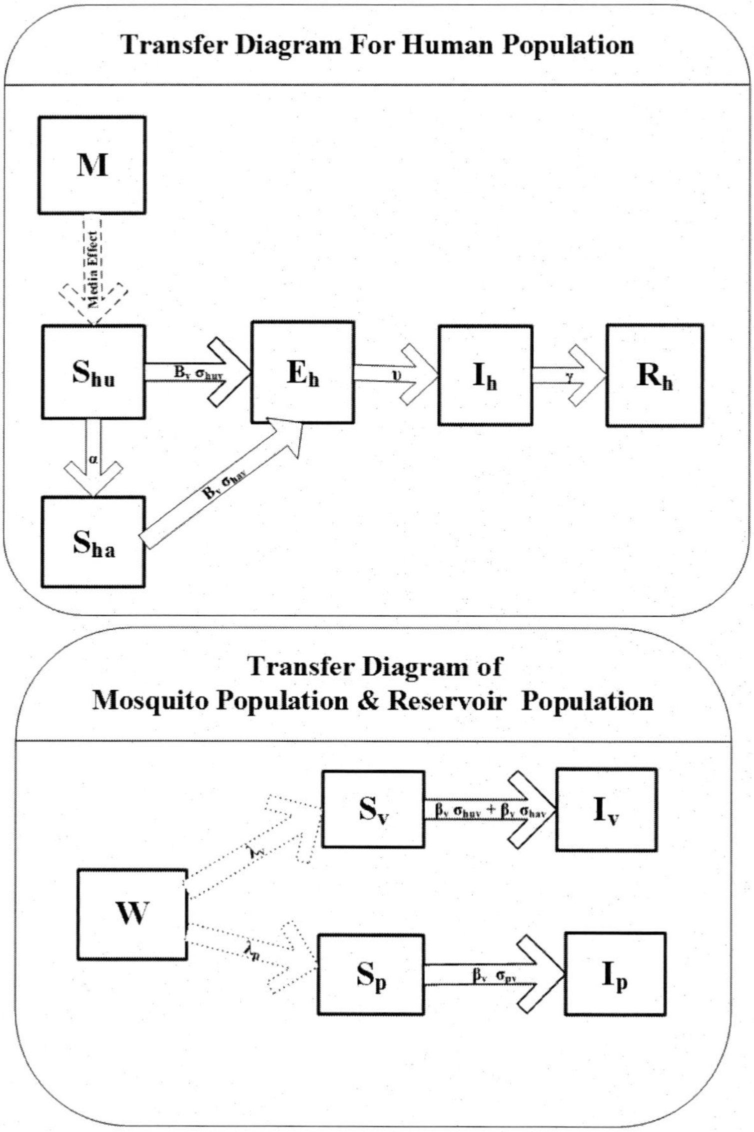

Figure 1. Transfer diagram.

Following rates of transfers and taking interaction of reservoir and mosquito population, mosquito and human population, the spread of Japanese Encephalitis is governed by the following system of non-linear differential equation.

$$\frac{dS_{hu}}{dt} = B_h - \alpha S_{hu} M - \beta_h \sigma_{huv} S_{hu} I_v - \mu_h S_{hu}$$

$$\frac{dS_{ha}}{dt} = \alpha S_{hu} M - \beta_h \sigma_{hav} S_{ha} I_v - \mu_h S_{ha}$$

$$\frac{dE_h}{dt} = \beta_h \sigma_{huv} S_{hu} I_v + \beta_h \sigma_{hav} S_{ha} I_v - (\mu_h + \nu) E_h$$

$$\frac{dI_h}{dt} = \nu E_h - (\gamma + \mu_h + \delta_h) I_h$$

$$\frac{dR_h}{dt} = \gamma I_h - \mu_h R_h$$

$$\frac{dS_v}{dt} = B_v + \lambda_v N_v W - \beta_v \sigma_{huv} S_v I_h - \beta_v \sigma_{hav} S_v I_h - \beta_v \sigma_{pv} P S_v - (\mu_v + \delta_v) S_v$$

$$\frac{dI_v}{dt} = \beta_v \sigma_{huv} S_v I_h + \beta_v \sigma_{hav} S_v I_h + \beta_v \sigma_{pv} P S_v - (\mu_v + \delta_v) I_v \qquad (1)$$

$$\frac{dS_p}{dt} = B_p + \lambda_p W N_p - (\mu_p + \delta_p) S_p - \beta_p \sigma_{pv} S_p I_v$$

$$\frac{dI_p}{dt} = \beta_p \sigma_{pv} S_p I_v - (\mu_p + \delta_p) I_p$$

$$\frac{dW}{dt} = B_e + \omega N_h - \theta W$$

$$\frac{dM}{dt} = \psi S_{hu} - \phi M$$

with, $N_h = S_{hu} + S_{ha} + E_h + I_h + R_h$,

$$N_v = S_v + I_v$$

$$N_p = S_p + I_p$$

and $S_{hu}, S_{ha}, E_h, R_h, S_v, S_p, W > 0$ and $I_h, I_v, I_p, M \geq 0$.

$$\frac{dN_h}{dt} = B_h - \mu_h N_h - \delta_h I_h$$

$$\frac{dN_h}{dt} \le B_h - \mu_h N_h \Rightarrow \lim_{t\to\infty} Sup N_h \le \frac{B_h}{\mu_h}$$

So, the possible region for the system is

$$\Lambda = \left\{ \begin{array}{l} (S_{hu}, S_{ha}, E_h, I_h, R_h, S_v, I_v, P, W, M) : (S_{hu}, S_{ha}, E_h, I_h, R_h) \le \frac{B_h}{\mu_h};\ 0 \le S_p \le \tilde{S}_p; \\ 0 \le W \le W_1;\ \ \&\ \ S_{hu}, S_{ha}, E_h, R_h, S_v, S_p, W > 0,\ I_h, I_v, I_p \ge 0,\ 0 \le M \le \tilde{M} \end{array} \right\}$$

Disease Free Equilibrium

Total rate of change of Human Population is

$$\frac{dN_h}{dt} = B_h - \mu_h N_h - \delta_h I_h$$

In the disease free equilibrium if we take rate of change of human population is zero, then

$$\frac{dN_h}{dt} \le B_h - \mu_h N_h \Rightarrow \lim_{t\to\infty} Sup N_h \le \frac{B_h}{\mu_h}$$

Let

$$E(S_{hu}, S_{ha}, E_h, I_h, R_h, S_v, I_v, S_p, I_p, W, M) = (S_{hu}, 0, 0, 0, 0, 0, 0, \tilde{S}_p, 0, W_1, \tilde{M})$$

then system of equation at the point gives

$$X_0 = (S_{hu}, 0, 0, 0, 0, 0, 0, \tilde{S}_p, 0, W_1, \tilde{M})$$

where $S_{hu} = \frac{B_h}{\mu_h}$,

$$N_h = S_{hu} + S_{ha} + E_h + I_h + R_h = \frac{B_h}{\mu_h} + 0 + 0 + 0 + 0 = \frac{B_h}{\mu_h}$$

$$W_1 = \frac{B_e + \omega N_h}{\theta} = \frac{B_e + \omega\left(\frac{B_h}{\mu_h}\right)}{\theta},\quad \tilde{S}_p = \left(\frac{B_p}{\mu_p + \delta_p - \lambda_p W_1}\right),\quad \tilde{M} = \frac{\Psi B_h}{\phi \mu_h}$$

So, we can see that there is a disease free equilibrium at $E_0(S_{hu}, S_{ha}, E_h, I_h, R_h, S_v, I_v, S_p, I_p, W, M)$

STABILITY OF DISEASE FREE EQUILIBRIUM

The disease free equilibrium is stable if all the eigenvalues of Jacobian of the system (1) have negative real parts. For this, the Jacobian of the system (1) at

$$E_0\left(S_{hu}, S_{ha}, E_h, I_h, R_h, S_v, I_v, S_p, I_p, W, M\right) = \left(\frac{B_h}{\mu_h}, 0,0,0,0,0,0,\hat{S}_p, 0, W_1, \tilde{M}\right)$$

is given by,

$$J_e = \begin{pmatrix} -\alpha\tilde{M}-\mu_h & 0 & 0 & 0 & 0 & 0 & -\beta_h\sigma_{huv}S_{hu} & 0 & 0 & 0 & -\alpha S_{hu} \\ \alpha\tilde{M} & -\mu_h & 0 & 0 & 0 & 0 & 0 & 0 & 0 & 0 & \alpha S_{hu} \\ 0 & 0 & -(\mu_h+\nu) & 0 & 0 & 0 & \beta_h\sigma_{huv}S_{hu} & 0 & 0 & 0 & 0 \\ 0 & 0 & \nu & -(\mu_h+\delta_h+\gamma) & 0 & 0 & 0 & 0 & 0 & 0 & 0 \\ 0 & 0 & 0 & \gamma & -\mu_h & 0 & 0 & 0 & 0 & 0 & 0 \\ 0 & 0 & 0 & 0 & 0 & \lambda_v W1-(\mu_v+\delta_v) & \lambda_v W1 & 0 & 0 & 0 & 0 \\ 0 & 0 & 0 & 0 & 0 & 0 & -(\mu_v+\delta_v) & 0 & 0 & 0 & 0 \\ 0 & 0 & 0 & 0 & 0 & 0 & -\beta_p\sigma_{pv}\tilde{S}_p & \lambda_p W1-(\mu_p+\delta_p) & \lambda_p W1 & \lambda_p\tilde{S}_p & 0 \\ 0 & 0 & 0 & 0 & 0 & 0 & \beta_p\sigma_{pv}\tilde{S}_p & 0 & -(\mu_p+\delta_p) & 0 & 0 \\ \omega & \omega & \omega & \omega & \omega & 0 & 0 & 0 & 0 & -\theta & 0 \\ \psi & 0 & 0 & 0 & 0 & 0 & 0 & 0 & 0 & 0 & -\phi \end{pmatrix}$$

Here, Trace of Jacobian matrix J_e is

$$Trace(J_e) = W_1\cdot\lambda_p - 2\cdot\delta_p - 2\cdot\delta_v - \gamma - 5\mu_h - 2\mu_p - 2\mu_v - \nu - \phi - \theta - M1\cdot\alpha - \delta_h + W_1\cdot\lambda_v$$

The disease free equilibrium is stable if all the eigenvalues of the Jacobian matrix of the system under consideration have negative real parts. Here, trace (J) is clearly negative. Now for Det (J_e), on solving we reach the relation $\lambda_v W_1 < \mu_v + \delta_v$ and $\lambda_p W_1 < \mu_p + \delta_p$. Here, $trace(J) < 0$ if $\lambda_v W_1 < \mu_v + \delta_v$ and

$$\det(J_e) = -\mu_h^2\cdot\theta\cdot(\delta_p+\mu_p)\cdot(\delta_v+\mu_v)\cdot(\mu_h+\nu)\cdot(\delta_p+\mu_p-W_1\cdot\lambda_p)\cdot(\delta_v+\mu_v-W_1\cdot\lambda_v)\cdot$$
$$(\delta_h+\mu_h+\gamma)\cdot(\mu_h\cdot\phi+M1\cdot\alpha\cdot\phi+S_{hu}\cdot\alpha\cdot\psi)$$
$$>0$$

This implies that the disease free equilibrium is locally asymptotically stable if $\lambda_v W_1 < \mu_v + \delta_v$ and $\lambda_p W_1 < \mu_p + \delta_p$ otherwise unstable.

NUMERICAL SIMULATION

To study the dynamical behavior of the model, numerical simulation of the system (1) is carried out using MATLAB12 using following rates.

Eigenvalues of Jacobian matrix J_e are -0.2600, -0.0001, -0.0150, -0.0594, -0.0186, -0.0150, -4.5370, -0.0159, -3.4000, -0.3000, -0.6000 negative if $\lambda_p W_1 < (\mu_p + \delta_p)$.

Table 2. Values of Variables and Parameters

Human Population	
B_h	150
μ_h	0.015
δ_h	0.022
β_h	0.3
σ_{huv}	0.011
σ_{hav}	0.011
v	0.0009
γ	4.5
α	0.0001
Mosquito Population	
B_v	600
λ_v	0.0001
μ_v	0.3
δ_v	0.3
β_v	0.3
Reservoir Population	
β_p	0.2
B_p	50
λ_p	0.000001
μ_p	0.1
δ_p	0.2
σ_{pv}	0.0011
Environment/Media	
W	20,000
M	30
ψ	0.005
ϕ	0.06
B_e	2
ω	0.0002
θ	0.0001

Trace of Jacobian matrix J_e is -2.4210 and determinant is 0.0000000000028539 it's also negative only if $\lambda_p W_1 < (\mu_p + \delta_p)$ and $\lambda_v W_1 < \mu_v + \delta_v$. This implies that the disease free equilibrium is locally asymptotically stable if $\lambda_p W_1 < (\mu_p + \delta_p)$ otherwise unstable.

MATLAB SIMULATION

This technique help us predict the future trends of an epidemic and thus help us be ready for future or take safety measures today for making a better future. Here, we take a sample population of 40,000. The results of simulation in different compartments are shown in following Figure 2-Figure 6:

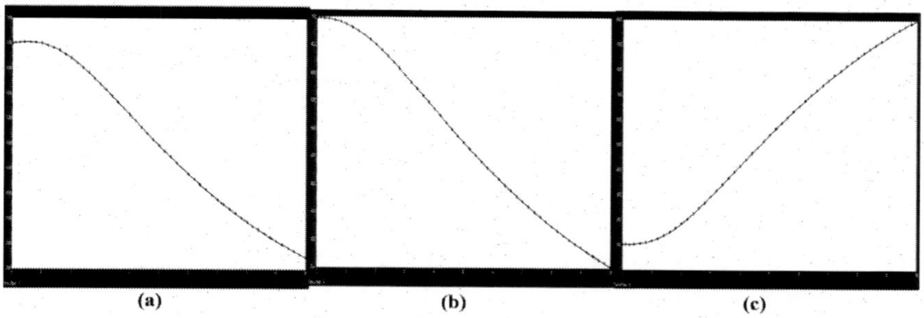

Figure 2. Human Population Dynamics in Different Compartments: (a) susceptible unaware; (b) susceptible aware; (c) human exposed.

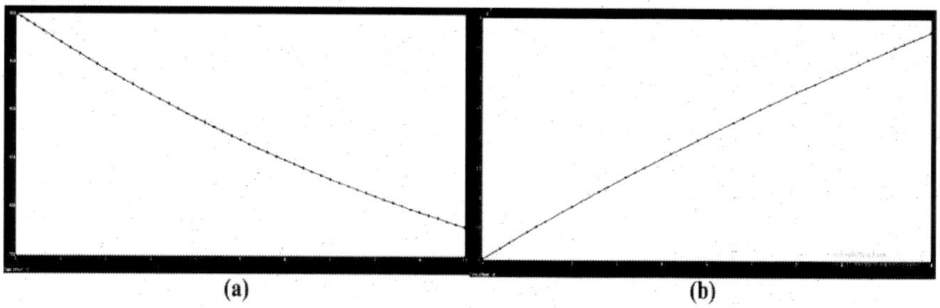

Figure 3. Human Population Dynamics in Different Compartments: (a) infected human; (b) recovered human.

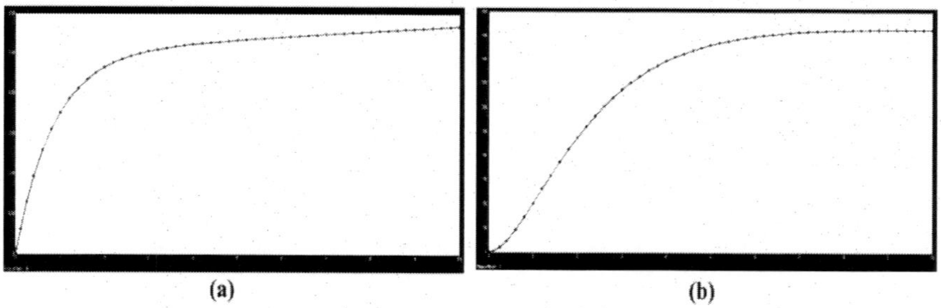

Figure 4. Mosquito Population Dynamics in Different Compartments: (a) susceptible mosquito; (b) infected mosquito.

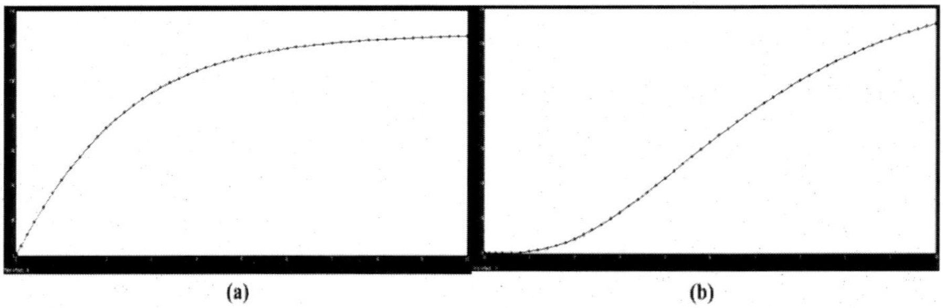

Figure 5. Reservoir Population Dynamics in Different Compartments: (a) susceptible reservoir; (b) infected reservoir.

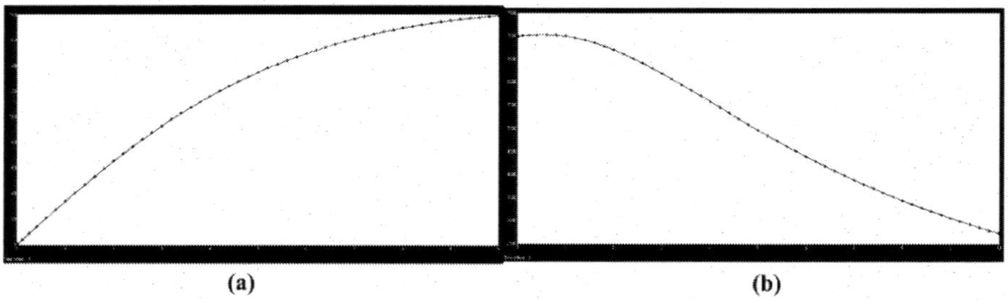

Figure 6. Effect of Media (a) and Environment (b).

In Figures 2 and 3, dynamics of human population in different compartments are shown. Susceptible unaware/aware are moves to exposed class exponentially in 10 days. Human exposure increases exponentially in 10 days. With awareness program through media, infected humans keep themselves isolated and helps to reduce the spread to 780 individuals in 10 days and hence removal from R_h - compartment increases uniformly in 10 days.

In Figure 4, dynamics of mosquito population is studied. It is shown that density in susceptible mosquito increases exponentially in first 3 days and thereafter almost at a constant rate. In first 5 days, susceptible mosquito get infected exponentially and thereafter at a constant rate. Similar are the observations for the susceptible reservoir and infectious reservoir (shown in Figure 5). So the target should be third day of the Japanese Encephalitis outbreak.

Figure 6 suggests that media is the powerful agent to aware the population about cleanliness and proper sanitation. The environment awareness will also help to stop the disease. It shows linear/uniform trend.

CONCLUSION

Here, we formulated a mathematical model using ordinary differential equations for Japanese Encephalitis. We divided the entire population into nine compartments and another two compartments are media and environmental discharges effect. Steady state conditions are derived which show that the disease free equilibrium is locally asymptotically stable only if.

Sensitivity analysis results tell us that we need to work more rigorously in order to control this epidemic. Numerical simulation is done using MATLAB 12.

ACKNOWLEDGMENT

The first author is very thankful to DST-FIST - file #MSI 097 for the financial assistance to carry out this research.

REFERENCES

[1] Gould, E. A. (2002). Flavivirus Infections in Humans. Encyclopedia of Life Sciences, Macmillan Publishers Ltd., *Nature Publishing group*, 220-244.

[2] Mukhopadhyay, B. B., Tapaswi, P. K., Chatterjee, A. and Mukherjee, B. (1993). A Mathematical Model for the Occurrences of Japanese Encephalitis. *Math. Comp. Model.*, 17, 99-103.

[3] Tapaswi, P. K., Ghosh, A. K. and Mukhopadhyay, B. B., (1995). Transmission of Japanese Encephalitis

[4] Naresh, R. Pandey, S. (2009). Modelling and analysis of the spread of Japanese Encephalitis with environmental effects, *Appl. Appl. Math.*, 4(1), 155-177.

In: Models and Methods for Supporting Decision-Making … ISBN: 978-1-63485-173-2
Editors: Carlos N. Bouza, Flávio L. de Mello et al.

Chapter 5

ESTIMATION AND COMPARISON OF THE LIKELIHOOD RATIOS OF BINARY DIAGNOSTIC TESTS

José Antonio Roldán-Nofuentes[1,*]
and Raid M. Amro[2,†]
[1]Department of Statistics (Biostatistics), Faculty of Medicine,
University of Granada, Granada, Spain
[2]Department of Mathematics, Faculty of Education,
Alquds Open University, Palestine

ABSTRACT

Positive and negative likelihood ratios are parameters that are used to assess and compare the accuracy of binary diagnostic tests. Likelihood ratios only depend on the sensitivity and specificity of the diagnostic test and quantify the increase in the knowledge about the presence of the disease through the application of the diagnostic test. This study is a review of likelihood ratios, their estimation for a single diagnostic test and the comparison of the likelihood ratios of two diagnostic tests in a paired design. Two programmes written in R are presented to solve the problems studied. The results are applied to the diagnosis of prostate cancer.

Keywords: binary diagnostic test, likelihood ratios, R software

INTRODUCTION

A diagnostic test is medical test that is applied to an individual in order to determine the presence or absence of a certain disease. The level of *PSA* for the diagnosis of prostate cancer and a stress test for the diagnosis of coronary artery disease are two examples of diagnostic

* E-mail: jaroldan@ugr.es.
† E-mail: ramro@qou.edu.

tests. The application of a diagnostic test (*DT*) for the assessment of diseases has different purposes [1]:

a) To provide reliable information about the disease status of an individual.
b) To influence the planning of the treatment of an individual.
c) To understand the mechanism and the nature of the disease through research.

The interpretation of a *DT* depends on several factors [1]:

a) On the intrinsic ability of the *DT* in order to distinguish between diseased and non-diseased individuals (discriminatory accuracy).
b) On the particular characteristics of each individual.
c) On the environment in which the *DT* is applied.

A *DT* may make a mistake in the diagnosis of the disease status of an individual, and therefore the accuracy of a *DT* is measured in terms of probabilities (or functions of them). When the result of a *DT* is positive (indicating the presence of the disease) or negative (indicating the absence of the disease), the *DT* is called a binary diagnostic test (*BDT*) and its accuracy is measured in terms of two fundamental parameters: sensitivity and specificity. Sensitivity (Se) is the probability of a positive result for the *BDT* when the individual has the disease, and specificity (Sp) is the probability of a negative result for the *BDT* when the individual does not have the disease. Other parameters to assess the performance of a *BDT* are the positive and negative likelihood ratios. The positive likelihood ratio (LR^{+}) is the ratio between the sensitivity and the probability of a positive result for the *BDT* when the individual does not have the disease $(1-Sp)$, and the negative likelihood ratio (LR^{-}) is the ratio between the probability of a negative result for the *BDT* when the patient has the disease $(1-Se)$ and the specificity. In order to obtain the unbiased estimators of the sensitivity and the specificity of the *BDT*, and therefore the likelihood ratios (*LRs*), it is necessary to know the true disease status (present or absent) of each individual in the random sample. The medical test through which the true disease status of each individual is known is called the gold standard (*GS*). A biopsy for the diagnosis of prostate cancer and an angiography for the diagnosis of coronary disease are two examples of *GSs*. Thus, there are two methods to diagnose the disease: *DT* and *GS*. The *DT* may make a mistake in the diagnosis of the disease while the *GS* does not. Why not always use the *GS*? There are several reasons to use a *DT* instead of a *GS*:

a) The *DT* is usually less expensive than the *GS*.
b) The use of a *GS* may lead to some risk for the individual. For example, a coronary angiography may cause a stroke, thrombosis or even the death of the individual.
c) There is not always a *GS*. For example, in the case of some psychiatric diseases.

The objective is to estimate the accuracy of the diagnosis, not to know if the individual has the disease or not.

LIKELIHOOD RATIOS OF A *BDT*

Let *D* be the random variable that models the result of the *GS*, in such a way that $D=1$ when the individual has the disease and $D=0$ when the individual does not have the disease. The probability $p=P(D=1)$ is the disease prevalence. Let *T* be the random variable that models the result of the *BDT*, in such a way that $T=1$ when the test result is positive (indicating the presence of the disease) and $T=0$ when the test result is negative (indicating the absence of the disease). The accuracy of the *BDT* is normally measured by the conditioned probabilities of correctly classifying a diseased and a non-diseased individual: sensitivity and specificity. Sensitivity is the probability of the *BDT* result being positive when the individual has the disease, i.e., $Se=P(T=1|D=1)$; and the specificity is the probability of the *BDT* result being negative when the individual does not have the disease, i.e., $Sp=P(T=0|D=0)$. The sensitivity and the specificity represent the accuracy of the *BDT* and only depend on its intrinsic ability to distinguish between diseased and non-diseased individuals. Both parameters depend on the biological, physical, chemical bases, etc... of the *BDT*. A *BDT* with high sensitivity is useful to exclude a diagnosis of the disease, and a *BDT* with high specificity is useful to confirm a diagnosis of the disease.

Other measurements of the performance of a *BDT* are the likelihood ratios (*LRs*) [2]. For a determined *BDT* result, the *LR* is the ratio between two probabilities, i.e.

$$LR=\frac{P(T=i|D=1)}{P(T=i|D=0)},\quad i=0,1.$$

When the *BDT* result is positive $(i=1)$, the *LR*, called the positive likelihood ratio (LR^{+}), is the ratio between the sensitivity and the probability of a positive *BDT* result when the individual does not have the disease, i.e.

$$LR^{+}=\frac{P(T=1|D=1)}{P(T=1|D=0)}=\frac{Se}{1-Sp}.$$

When the *BDT* result is negative $(i=0)$, the *LR*, called the negative likelihood ratio (LR^{-}), is the ratio between the probability of a negative *BDT* result when the individual has the disease and the specificity, i.e.

$$LR^{-}=\frac{P(T=0|D=1)}{P(T=0|D=0)}=\frac{1-Se}{Sp}.$$

The likelihood ratios only depend on the sensitivity and the specificity of the diagnostic test, and their values vary between zero and infinity. When the *BDT* and the *GS* are independent then $LR^{+}=LR^{-}=1$, and if the *BDT* correctly classifies all of the individuals (with or without the disease) then $LR^{+}=\infty$ and $LR^{-}=0$. A value of $LR^{+}>1$ indicates that a positive *BDT* result is more probable for an individual who has the disease than for one who does not, and a value of $LR^{-}<1$ indicates that a negative *BDT* result is more probable for an individual who does not have the disease than for one who does. The likelihood ratios quantify the increase in knowledge of the presence of the disease through the application of the *BDT*. Before applying the *BDT*, the odds of an individual having the disease is

$$\text{pre-test odds } = \frac{p}{1-p},$$

and after applying the *BDT* the odds of an individual having the disease are

$$\text{post-test odds} = \frac{P(D=1|T=i)}{P(D=0|T=i)},\ i=0,1\ .$$

Likelihood ratios relate the pre-test odds to the post-tests odds, i.e.

$$\text{Post-test odds } (T=1) = LR^{+} \times \text{pre-test odds}$$
$$\text{Post-test odds } (T=0) = LR^{-} \times \text{pre-test odds,}$$

and, therefore, the likelihood ratios quantify the change in the odds of the disease obtained through the knowledge of the application of the *BDT*. Now it's presented the estimation of the *LRs* of a *BDT* subject to a cross-sectional study and subject to a case-control study.

ESTIMATION OF THE *LRS* OF A *BDT*

The estimation of the *LRs* can be carried out through a cross-sectional study or through a case-control study. In a cross-sectional study, the *BDT* and the *GS* are applied to all of the individuals in a random sample sized *n*; and in a case-control study, the *BDT* is applied to all of the individuals in two samples, one of n_1 individuals who have the disease and another of n_2 who do not have the disease.

Table 1. Observed frequencies in a cross-sectional study

	$T=1$	$T=0$	Total
$D=1$	s_1	s_0	s
$D=0$	r_1	r_0	r
Total	s_1+r_1	s_0+r_0	n

Estimation Subject to a Cross-Sectional Study

The frequencies given in Table 1 are obtained when the *BDT* and the *GS* are applied to all of the individuals in a random sample sized n (cross-sectional study). In this table, s_i is the number of individuals in which $T=i$ and $D=1$, r_i is the number of individuals in which $T=i$ and $D=0$ (with $i=0,1$), $s=s_1+s_0$, $r=r_1+r_0$ and $n=s+r$. The maximum likelihood estimators of the *LRs* are

$$LR^+=\frac{s_1 r}{r_1 s} \text{ and } LR^-=\frac{s_0 r}{r_0 s},$$

and applying the Delta method [3] their estimated variances are

$$Var\left(LR^+\right)\approx\frac{\left(1-\hat{S}e\right)LR^+}{s\left(1-\hat{S}p\right)}+\frac{\hat{S}p\left(1-\hat{S}p\right)\left(LR^+\right)^2}{r\left(1-\hat{S}p\right)^2}$$

and

$$Var\left(LR^-\right)\approx\frac{\hat{S}eLR^-}{s\hat{S}p}+\frac{\hat{S}p\left(1-\hat{S}p\right)\left(LR^-\right)^2}{r\hat{S}p^2},$$

where $\hat{S}e=s_1/s$ and $\hat{S}p=r_0/r$ are the estimators of the sensitivity and the specificity respectively. Conditioning in the disease status (*GS*), the *LRs* are technically equivalent to a relative risk and, therefore, their estimation consists of the estimation of a relative risk. Martín-Andrés and Álvarez-Hernández [4] studied confidence intervals (*CIs*) for the ratio of two independent binomial proportions (as is the case with the relative risk). Adapting the results of these authors to the notation in Table 1, the *CIs* for the *LRs* are

$$LR^+\in\frac{n's_1'r_1'+\frac{z_{1-\alpha/2}^2}{2}\left(s's_1'+r'r_1'-2s_1'r_1'\right)\pm z_{1-\alpha/2}\sqrt{n'^2s_1'r_1'\left(s_1'+r_1'-n'\hat{p}_1'\hat{p}_2'\right)+\frac{z_{1-\alpha/2}^2}{4}\left(s's_1'-r'r_1'\right)^2}}{r_1'\left\{n's'\hat{p}_1'-z_{1-\alpha/2}^2\left(s'-r_1'\right)\right\}}$$

and

$$LR^-\in\frac{n's_0'r_0'+\frac{z_{1-\alpha/2}^2}{2}\left(s's_0'+r'r_0'-2s_0'r_0'\right)\pm z_{1-\alpha/2}\sqrt{n'^2s_0'r_0'\left(s_0'+r_0'-n'\hat{p}_3'\hat{p}_4'\right)+\frac{z_{1-\alpha/2}^2}{4}\left(s's_0'-r'r_0'\right)^2}}{r_0'\left\{n's'\hat{p}_3'-z_{1-\alpha/2}^2\left(s'-r_0'\right)\right\}}$$

where $s_i' = s_i + 0.5$, $r_i' = r_i + 0.5$, $s' = s_1' + s_0'$, $r' = r_1' + r_0'$, $n' = s' + r'$, $\hat{p}_1' = r_1'/r'$, $\hat{p}_2' = s_1'/s'$, $\hat{p}_3' = r_0'/r'$ and $\hat{p}_4' = s_0'/s'$. If the upper limit of the interval for the LR^+ is lower than $s_1'/(n' - r_1')$ or higher than $\overset{+}{LR}$, then the upper limit of the interval is

$$\frac{1}{s'\left(\hat{p}_1'\right)^2 + z_{1-\alpha/2}^2}\left\{s_1'\hat{p}_1' + \frac{z_{1-\alpha/2}^2}{2} - z_{1-\alpha/2}\sqrt{\frac{z_{1-\alpha/2}^2}{4} + s_1'\left(\hat{p}_1' - \hat{p}_2'\right)}\right\},$$

and the upper limit of this interval is higher than $(n' - s_1')/r_1'$ or lower than $\overset{-}{LR}$, then the upper limit of the interval is

$$\frac{1}{r'\left(\hat{p}_1'\right)^2}\left\{r_1'\hat{p}_2' + \frac{z_{1-\alpha/2}^2}{2} + z_{1-\alpha/2}\sqrt{\frac{z_{1-\alpha/2}^2}{4} + r_1'\left(\hat{p}_2' - \hat{p}_1'\right)}\right\}.$$

Regarding the *CI* for LR^-, if the upper limit of this interval is lower than $s_0'/(n' - r_0')$ or higher than $\overset{-}{LR}$, then the lower limit of the interval is

$$\frac{1}{s'\left(\hat{p}_3'\right)^2 + z_{1-\alpha/2}^2}\left\{s_0'\hat{p}_3' + \frac{z_{1-\alpha/2}^2}{2} - z_{1-\alpha/2}\sqrt{\frac{z_{1-\alpha/2}^2}{4} + s_0'\left(\hat{p}_3' - \hat{p}_4'\right)}\right\},$$

and if the upper limit of this interval is higher than $(n' - s_0')/r_0'$ or lower than $\overset{-}{LR}$, then the upper limit of the interval is

$$\frac{1}{r'\left(\hat{p}_3'\right)^2}\left\{r_0'\hat{p}_4' + \frac{z_{1-\alpha/2}^2}{2} + z_{1-\alpha/2}\sqrt{\frac{z_{1-\alpha/2}^2}{4} + r_0'\left(\hat{p}_4' - \hat{p}_3'\right)}\right\}.$$

In the URL “http://www.ugr.es/~bioest/software/cmd.php?seccion=mdb” there is a programme in R [5] to estimate the *LRs* of a *BDT* subject to a cross-sectional study. This programme, called “elrbdt” (estimation of the *LRs* of a *BDT*), runs with the command "elrbdt(s_1, s_0, r_1, r_0)" when the confidence level of the intervals is 95%, and with the command "elrbdt$(s_1, s_0, r_1, r_0, \mathit{conflevel})$" when the confidence level is $(100 \times \mathit{conflevel})\%$.

Estimation Subject to a Case-Control Study

When the design is case-control (the *BDT* is applied to two independent samples, one of n_1 individuals who have the disease and another one of n_2 individuals who do not have the disease), the results given in Section 3.1 are valid substituting s with n_1 and r with n_2 (Table 2). The programme "elrbdt" is valid in a case-control study.

Table 2. Observed frequencies in a case-control study

	$T=1$	$T=0$	Total
$D=1$	s_1	s_0	n_1
$D=0$	r_1	r_0	n_2
Total	s_1+r_1	s_0+r_0	n

Application to the Diagnosis of Prostate Cancer

Prostate cancer is one of the most frequent cancers among men and its diagnosis can be made through the *PSA* test, and a biopsy is used as the gold standard. Roberts et al. [6] have studied the diagnosis of prostate cancer in 1280 men using the *PSA* and the biopsy. The results of Robert et al. [6] are shown in Table 3. Using the "elrbdt" programme and running the command "elrbdt$(395,76,472,337)$" it holds that $LR^+ = 1.437$ and $LR^- = 0.387$, and the respective standard errors are 0.052 and 0.044. The 95% *CIs* of Martín-Andrés and Alvarez-Hernández [4] for the *LRs* are:

$$LR^+ \in (1.337\ ;\ 1.540) \quad \text{and} \quad LR^- \in (0.309\ ;\ 0.482)$$

Therefore, the probability of the *PSA* test being positive for individuals who have prostate cancer is a value between 1.337 and 1.540 times higher than the probability of the *PSA* test being positive for individuals who do not have prostate cancer, with a confidence level of 95%. The probability of the *PSA* test being negative for individuals who do not have prostate cancer is a value between 2.075 $(=1/0.482)$ and 3.236 $(=1/0.309)$ times higher than the probability of that test being negative for individuals who have prostate cancer, with a confidence level of 95%.

Table 3. Observed frequencies in the study by Roberts et al. [6]

	$T=1$	$T=0$	Total
$D=1$	395	76	471
$D=0$	472	337	809
Total	867	413	1280

COMPARISON OF THE *LRs* OF TWO *BDTs*

The comparison of the performance of two *BDTs* is an important topic in the field of Statistical Methods in Medical Sciences and has been the subject of numerous studies in statistical literature. The most common situation to compare the performance of two *BDTs* is a paired design. This type of design consists of applying the two *BDTs* and the *GS* to all of the individuals in a random sample sized *n*. Now it's presented the comparison of the *LRs* of two *BDTs* subject to a paired design.

Comparison Subject to a Paired Design

The comparison of the *LRs* of two *BDTs* subject to a paired design has been the subject of several studies. Leisenring and Pepe [7] studied the estimation and the comparison of the *LRs* of two *BDTs* through *GEE* models. Roldán Nofuentes et al. [8] studied the comparison of the *LRs* of two binary tests through the method of maximum likelihood and compared their results with those of Leisenring and Pepe [7], and found that both methods give very similar results (in terms of type I error and power). Dolgun et al. [9] extended the results of Leisenring and Pepe [7] and proposed a *GEE* model to simultaneously compare the *LRs* of two *BDTs*. Now it's presented of Roldán-Nofuentes et al. [8].

Let T_1 and T_2 be the random variables that model the results of the *BDTs* 1 and 2 respectively, in such a way that $T_i = 1$ when the result of the *i-th* test is positive and $T_i = 0$ when the result is negative $(i = 1,2)$. Let *D* be the random variable that models the disease status ($D = 1$ when the individual has the disease and $D = 0$ when the individual does not have the disease). Let $Se_i = P(T_i = 1|D = 1)$ and $Sp_i = P(T_i = 0|D = 0)$ be the sensitivity and the specificity of the *i-th BDT*. The application of the two *BDTs* and the *GS* to all of the individuals in a random sample sized *n* gives rise to Table 4, where s_{ij} is the number of individuals in which $T_1 = i$, $T_2 = j$ and $D = 1$, with $i, j = 0,1$, r_{ij} is the number of individuals in which $T_1 = i$, $T_2 = j$ and $D = 0$, $s = \sum_{i,j=0}^{1} s_{ij}$, $r = \sum_{i,j=0}^{1} r_{ij}$ and $n = s + r$.

The data in Table 4 are the product of a multinomial distribution whose probabilities are shown in Table 5. When the results of the two *BDTs* are positive the hypothesis test to check the equality of the *LRs* is

$$H_0 : \omega^+ = 0 \text{ vs } H_1 : \omega^+ \neq 0,$$

and when the results of both *BDTs* are negative the hypothesis test is

$$H_0 : \omega^- = 0 \text{ vs } H_1 : \omega^- \neq 0,$$

where $\omega^+ = \ln\left(LR_1^+ / LR_2^+\right)$ and $\omega^- = \ln\left(LR_1^- / LR_2^-\right)$.

Table 4. Observed frequencies subject to a paired design

	$T_1 = 1$		$T_1 = 0$		
	$T_2 = 1$	$T_2 = 0$	$T_2 = 1$	$T_2 = 0$	Total
$D = 1$	s_{11}	s_{10}	s_{01}	s_{00}	s
$D = 0$	r_{11}	r_{10}	r_{01}	r_{00}	r
Total	$s_{11} + r_{11}$	$s_{10} + r_{10}$	$s_{01} + r_{01}$	$s_{00} + r_{00}$	n

Table 5. Probabilities subject to a paired design

	$T_1 = 1$		$T_1 = 0$		
	$T_2 = 1$	$T_2 = 0$	$T_2 = 1$	$T_2 = 0$	Total
$D = 1$	p_{11}	p_{10}	p_{01}	p_{00}	p
$D = 0$	q_{11}	q_{10}	q_{01}	q_{00}	q
Total	$p_{11} + q_{11}$	$p_{10} + q_{10}$	$p_{01} + q_{01}$	$p_{00} + q_{00}$	1

In terms of the probabilities given in Table 5, the positive *LRs* are written as

$$LR_1^+ = \frac{1-p}{p} \frac{p_{11} + p_{10}}{q_{11} + q_{10}} \quad \text{and} \quad LR_2^+ = \frac{1-p}{p} \frac{p_{11} + p_{01}}{q_{11} + q_{01}},$$

and the negative *LRs* as

$$LR_1^- = \frac{1-p}{p} \frac{p_{01} + p_{00}}{q_{01} + q_{00}} \quad \text{and} \quad LR_2^- = \frac{1-p}{p} \frac{p_{10} + p_{00}}{q_{10} + q_{00}},$$

where $p = \sum_{i,j=0}^{1} p_{ij}$ is the disease prevalence and $q = 1 - p = \sum_{i,j=0}^{1} q_{ij}$. In this way, it holds that

$$\omega^+ = \ln\left\{\frac{(p_{11} + p_{10})(q_{11} + q_{01})}{(p_{11} + p_{01})(q_{11} + q_{10})}\right\} \quad \text{and} \quad \omega^- = \ln\left\{\frac{(p_{01} + p_{00})(q_{10} + q_{00})}{(p_{10} + p_{00})(q_{01} + q_{00})}\right\}.$$

Let $\boldsymbol{\pi} = (p_{00}, p_{01}, p_{10}, p_{11}, q_{00}, q_{01}, q_{10}, q_{11})^T$ be a vector whose components are the probabilities in Table 5. As the probabilities p_{ij} and q_{ij} are probabilities of a multinomial distribution, their maximum likelihood estimators are

$$\hat{p}_{ij} = \frac{s_{ij}}{n_{ij}} \quad \text{and} \quad \hat{q}_{ij} = \frac{n_{ij}}{n},$$

and the estimated variance-covariance matrix of $\hat{\boldsymbol{\pi}}$ is $\hat{\Sigma}_{\hat{\boldsymbol{\pi}}} = \left\{ \text{diag}\left(\hat{\boldsymbol{\pi}}\right) - \hat{\boldsymbol{\pi}}\hat{\boldsymbol{\pi}}^T \right\} / n$. The maximum likelihood estimators of the positive *LRs* are

$$\hat{LR}_1^+ = \frac{r\left(s_{11} + s_{10}\right)}{s\left(r_{11} + r_{10}\right)} \text{ and } \hat{LR}_2^+ = \frac{r\left(s_{11} + s_{01}\right)}{s\left(r_{11} + r_{01}\right)},$$

and maximum likelihood estimators of the negative *LRs* are

$$\hat{LR}_1^- = \frac{r\left(s_{01} + s_{00}\right)}{s\left(r_{01} + r_{00}\right)} \text{ and } \hat{LR}_2^- = \frac{r\left(s_{10} + s_{00}\right)}{s\left(r_{10} + r_{00}\right)}.$$

Then the maximum likelihood estimators of ω^+ and ω^- are

$$\hat{\omega}^+ = \ln\left\{ \frac{\left(s_{11} + s_{10}\right)\left(r_{11} + r_{01}\right)}{\left(s_{11} + s_{01}\right)\left(r_{11} + r_{10}\right)} \right\} \text{ and } \hat{\omega}^- = \ln\left\{ \frac{\left(s_{01} + s_{00}\right)\left(r_{10} + r_{00}\right)}{\left(s_{10} + s_{00}\right)\left(r_{01} + r_{00}\right)} \right\},$$

and applying the Delta method [3] the estimated variance of ω is

$$\hat{Var}\left(\hat{\omega}\right) \approx \left(\frac{\partial \omega}{\partial \boldsymbol{\pi}}\right)_{\boldsymbol{\pi}=\hat{\boldsymbol{\pi}}} \hat{\Sigma}_{\hat{\boldsymbol{\pi}}} \left(\frac{\partial \omega}{\partial \boldsymbol{\pi}}\right)^T_{\boldsymbol{\pi}=\hat{\boldsymbol{\pi}}},$$

where ω is ω^+ or ω^-. Finally, the statistic for the hypothesis test $H_0 : \omega = 0$ vs $H_1 : \omega \neq 0$ is

$$z = \frac{\hat{\omega}}{\sqrt{\hat{Var}\left(\hat{\omega}\right)}} \xrightarrow[n\to\infty]{} N\left(0,1\right).$$

Moreover, an asymptotic *CI* for ω is

$$\omega \in \hat{\omega} \pm z_{1-\alpha/2}\sqrt{\hat{Var}\left(\hat{\omega}\right)},$$

where $z_{1-\alpha/2}$ is the $100\left(1-\alpha/2\right)th$ percentile of the normal standard distribution. The *CI* for the ratio of the two positive (negative) *LRs* is obtained by taking the exponential, i.e.

$$\frac{LR_1}{LR_2} \in \exp\left\{ \hat{\omega} \pm z_{1-\alpha/2}\sqrt{\hat{Var}\left(\hat{\omega}\right)} \right\}.$$

Roldán-Nofuentes et al. [8] also studied the simultaneous comparison of the *LRs* of the two *BDTs*. The previous hypothesis tests compare the naperian logarithms of the positive and negative *LRs* in an independent manner. Nevertheless, the positive *LR* and the negative *LR* of each *BDT* depend on the same parameters (the sensitivity and specificity of each diagnostic test) and, therefore, it is possible to study the simultaneous comparison of both parameters. This hypothesis test consists of solving the global hypothesis test

$$H_0:\left(\omega^- = 0 \text{ and } \omega^+ = 0\right) \text{ vs } H_1:\left(\omega^- \neq 0 \text{ and/or } \omega^+ \neq 0\right).$$

Applying the central theorem of the multivariate limit it holds that

$$\sqrt{n}\begin{pmatrix}\hat{\omega}^+ - \omega^+ \\ \hat{\omega}^- - \omega^-\end{pmatrix} \xrightarrow[n\to\infty]{} N\left[\mu = \begin{pmatrix}0\\0\end{pmatrix}, \Sigma_{\pi} = \begin{pmatrix}\sigma_{11} & \sigma_{12}\\ \sigma_{12} & \sigma_{22}\end{pmatrix}\right],$$

where the elements of the variance-covariance matrix are estimated applying the Delta method [3]. In this way, if $\boldsymbol{\omega} = \left(\omega^+, \omega^-\right)^T$ then

$$\hat{\Sigma}_{\hat{\boldsymbol{\omega}}} \approx \left(\frac{\partial \boldsymbol{\omega}}{\partial \boldsymbol{\pi}}\right)_{\boldsymbol{\pi}=\hat{\boldsymbol{\pi}}} \hat{\Sigma}_{\hat{\boldsymbol{\pi}}} \left(\frac{\partial \boldsymbol{\omega}}{\partial \boldsymbol{\pi}}\right)^T_{\boldsymbol{\pi}=\hat{\boldsymbol{\pi}}},$$

and the test statistic of the global hypothesis test is

$$Q^2 = \hat{\boldsymbol{\omega}}^T \overset{-1}{\Sigma}_{\hat{\boldsymbol{\omega}}} \hat{\boldsymbol{\omega}} \xrightarrow[n\to\infty]{} \chi^2_2 .$$

Finally, the comparison of the *LRs* of the two *BDTs* subject to a paired design is realized following the next steps: 1) Solve the global hypothesis test $H_0:\left(\omega^- = 0 \text{ and } \omega^+ = 0\right)$ to an error of α using the statistic $Q^2 = \hat{\boldsymbol{\omega}}^T \overset{-1}{\Sigma}_{\hat{\boldsymbol{\omega}}} \hat{\boldsymbol{\omega}}$; 2) If the global hypothesis test is not significant to an error of α, then the homogeneity of the *LRs* of the two *BDTs* is not rejected, but if the global hypothesis test is significant to an error of α, then the study of the causes of the significance is performed by solving hypothesis tests $H_0:\omega^+ = 0$ and $H_0:\omega^- = 0$ along with a multiple comparison method (e.g., Bonferroni [10], Holm [11] or Hochberg [12], which are methods that are very easy to apply) to an error of α.

In the URL "http://www.ugr.es/~bioest/software/cmd.php?seccion=mdb" there is a programme in R [5] to compare the *LRs* of a *BDT* subject to a paired design. This programme, called "clrpd" (comparison of the *LRs* subject to a paired design), runs with the command "clrpd$\left(s_{11}, s_{10}, s_{01}, s_{00}, r_{11}, r_{10}, r_{01}, r_{00}\right)$" when the hypothesis tests are solved to an error of $\alpha = 5\%$, and with the command "clrpd$\left(s_{11}, s_{10}, s_{01}, s_{00}, r_{11}, r_{10}, r_{01}, r_{00}, \alpha\right)$" when the hypothesis tests are solved to an error of $\alpha\%$. The programme first solves the global hypothesis test and then the individual hypothesis tests. It also calculates the confidence intervals for ω and for the ratio of the two positive (negative) *LRs*.

Application to the Diagnosis of Prostate Cancer

Prostate cancer can also be diagnosed through a physical test known as a rectal examination. Roberts et al. [6] also applied this test to the sample of 1280 men. The results of Robert et al. [6] are shown in Table 6, where variable T_1 models the result of the *PSA*, the variable T_2 models that of the rectal examination and the variable *D* the result of the biopsy. Using the "clrpd" programme and running the command "clrpd$(229,166,60,16,144,328,267,70)$" it holds that $\overset{+}{LR_1} = 1.437$, $\overset{-}{LR_1} = 0.387$, $\overset{+}{LR_2} = 1.208$ and $\overset{-}{LR_2} = 0.785$, and their respective standard errors are 0.052, 0.044, 0.061 and 0.054. Furthermore, $\hat{\omega}^+ = 0.174$ and $\hat{\omega}^- = -0.707$, and the estimated variance-covariance matrix of $\hat{\boldsymbol{\omega}} = \left(\hat{\omega}^+, \hat{\omega}^-\right)^T$ is

$$\hat{\Sigma}_{\hat{\boldsymbol{\omega}}} \approx \begin{pmatrix} 0.005 & -0.009 \\ -0.009 & 0.021 \end{pmatrix}.$$

Table 6. Observed frequencies in the study by Roberts et al. [6]

	$T_1 = 1$		$T_1 = 0$		
	$T_2 = 1$	$T_2 = 0$	$T_2 = 1$	$T_2 = 0$	Total
$D = 1$	229	166	60	16	471
$D = 0$	144	328	267	70	809
Total	373	494	327	86	1280

The statistic for the global hypothesis test is $Q^2 = 34.83$ $\left(\text{p-value} = 2.73 \times 10^{-8}\right)$, and therefore the global hypothesis test of equality of the likelihood ratios of the two diagnostic tests is rejected. Applying the marginal hypothesis tests, the value of the statistic for the test $H_0 : \omega^+ = 0$ is $z = 2.450$ $\left(\text{two-sided p-value} = 0.014\right)$, and the value of the statistic for the the test $H_0 : \omega^- = 0$ is $z = 4.904$ $\left(\text{two-sided p-value} = 9.37 \times 10^{-7}\right)$. In order to study the causes of the significance of the global hypothesis test, a multiple comparison method is applied. Applying the method of Bonferroni [10], Holm [11] or Hochberg [12], to an error of $\alpha = 5\%$, the two hypotheses $H_0 : \omega^+ = 0$ and $H_0 : \omega^- = 0$ are rejected. From the results the following conclusions are obtained:

a) The 95% *CI* for $\dfrac{LR_1^+}{LR_2^+}$ is (1.035; 1.368), and therefore the positive likelihood ratio of the *PSA* is significantly greater than positive likelihood ratio of the rectal examination.

b) The 95% *CI* for $\frac{LR_1^-}{LR_2^-}$ is (0.372; 0.654), and therefore the negative likelihood ratio of the *PSA* is significantly lower than the negative likelihood ratio of the rectal examination.

Conclusion

Along with sensitivity and specificity, likelihood ratios are one of the most widely used measurements to evaluate and compare the performance of *BDTs*, and the information they provide, and in clinical terms they represent very useful measurements to evaluate and compare the quality of *BDTs*.

The *LRs* have three properties which make them more useful that other parameters of a diagnostic test (e.g., predictive values): a) the *LRs* do not depend on disease prevalence; b) the *LRs* can be calculated for diagnostic tests with more than two levels; c) and *LRs* allow to assess the impact of a diagnostic test result on the probability of a patient being diseased. The *LRs* only depend on the intrinsic ability of the diagnostic test to distinguish between a diseased patient and a non-diseased one, and therefore the *LRs* are superior measurements of the performance of *BDTs*.

This study is a review of *LRs*, their estimation for a *BDT* and the comparison of the *LRs* of two *BDTs* in a paired design. Two R programmes to solve the problems studied are available in the URL "http://www.ugr.es/~bioest/software/cmd.php?seccion=mdb."

Acknowledgment

This research was supported by the Spanish Ministry of Science, Grant Number MTM2012-35591. We thank the Prof. Carlos Bouza and the other editors their efforts and interest in this book. We thank the two referees for their helpful comments that improved the quality of this chapter.

References

[1] Zhou X. H., Obuchowski N. A., McClish D. K., 2002. Statistical methods in diagnostic medicine. Wiley, New York.

[2] Pepe, M. S., 2003 The statistical evaluation of medical tests for classification and prediction. Oxford University Press, New York.

[3] Agresti, A., 2002. Categorical data analysis. John Wiley and Sons, New York.

[4] Martín-Andrés A., Álvarez-Hernández M., 2014. Two-tailed approximate confidence intervals for the ratio of proportions. *Statistics and Computing,* 24, 65-75.

[5] R. Development Core Team. R: A language and environment for statistical computing. R Foundation for Statistical Computing, Vienna, Austria. ISBN 3-900051-07-0, 2011, URL http://www.R-project.org.

[6] Roberts, R. O., Bergstralh, E. J., Lieber, M. M., Jacobsen, S. J., 2000. Digital rectal examination and prostate-specific antigen abnormalities at the time of prostate biopsy and biopsy outcomes, 1980 to 1997. *Urology,* 56, 817-822.

[7] Leisenring W., Pepe M. S., 1998. Regression modelling of diagnostic likelihood ratios for the evaluation of medical diagnostic tests. *Biometrics,* 54, 444-442.

[8] Roldán-Nofuentes, J. A., Luna del Castillo, J. D., 2007. Comparison of the likelihood ratios of two binary diagnostic tests in paired designs. *Statistics in Medicine,* 26, 4179-4201.

[9] Dolgun N. A., Harika Gozukara H., Karaagaoglu E., 2012. Comparing diagnostic tests: test of hypothesis for likelihood ratios. *Journal of Statistical Computation and Simulation,* 82, 369-381.

[10] Bonferroni, C. E., 1936. Teoria statistica delle classi e calcolo delle probabilità. *Pubblicazioni del R Istituto Superiore di Scienze Economiche e Commerciali di Firenze,* 8, 3-62.

[11] Holm, S., 1979. A simple sequential rejective multiple testing procedure. *Scandinavian Journal of Statistics,* 6, 65-70.

[12] Hochberg, Y., 1988. A sharper Bonferroni procedure for multiple tests of significance. *Biometrika,* 75, 800-802.

In: Models and Methods for Supporting Decision-Making … ISBN: 978-1-63485-173-2
Editors: Carlos N. Bouza, Flávio L. de Mello et al.

Chapter 6

HEALTH PLANNING INFORMATION ACQUIRED FROM UNSTRUCTURED DATA ABOUT DIABETES MELLITUS

Rodrigo Santos Souza[1], Edilberto Strauss[2] and Flávio Luis de Mello[2,*]

[1]State University of Ceará and Federal Institute of Ceará, CE, Brazil
[2]Electronic and Computer Engineering Department,
Federal University of Rio de Janeiro,
Rio de Janeiro, Brazil

ABSTRACT

This chapter presents a work on the usage of the crowd's knowledge, the application of semantics in the context of the Internet, and the social networking phenomenon in order to provide a collaborative information platform applied to health planning. A proof of concept was developed based on diabetes disease, providing a description of the methodology employed and the fundamentals aspect that support this study. The exponential growth of Internet content suggests that there is an opportunity for developing a more selective and qualitative knowledge consume. It might be adapted to population' health improvement and disease prevention. On the Internet, and more specifically on social networks, blogs and other forms of expression, such health knowledge is spread into the crowd, where information is provided in a collaborative way. Therefore, this work aims to investigate the current situation of dispersed knowledge over the Internet and use it to support strategic planning within the Brazilian public health.

Keywords: social networks, information retrieval, public health, Internet 2.0

* E-mail: flavioluis.mello@gmail.com.

INTRODUCTION

This work studies the use of crowd's knowledge, the application of semantics in the context of the Internet and the social networking phenomenon as a collaborative information platform applied to health planning. The proposed proof of concept concerns the diabetes mellitus. The evidence-based medicine methodology called PICO (patient, intervention, comparison and outcomes) is used to acquire the existing knowledge. This study can be applied to different diseases or other aspects related to population health, where documents seek and messages analysis over social networks can provide complementarily clinical evidences. The methodology presented here can also be used in other sources of unstructured or semi-structured data such as HIS (Health Information Systems) and its variations, and can be even applied to the physical records once converted to digital textual data.

Health plan is an extremely difficult task and requires wide perspective over the organization, the population's needs, provided services, membership opportunities, continuity and services expansion. Brazilian managers have standardized the coverage and planning tools of Health Planning through the guidelines and methodology provided by PlanejaSUS, a Ministry of Health program. Therefore, decision makers organize their efforts based on technical and policy guidance.

At the initial phase of planning, called situational assessment, managers observe parameters and past indicators, studying the results, creating timeline visions to support the next steps in the planning and management cycle. At this stage, it is quite common to use the SUS (Sistema Único de Saúde – Single Health System) information systems and public data as well as decision support tools based on business intelligence, and some more technologically sophisticated data mining tools from Brazilian districts. This data collection is necessary in order to guide the process of strategic health planning, to identify problems and opportunities, and to improve and expand the planning actions. However, a value added service can be obtained.

The exponential growth of Internet content suggests that there is an opportunity for developing a more selective and qualitative knowledge consume. It is known that on the Internet, and more specifically on social networks, blogs and other forms of expression, such knowledge is spread into the crowds, where information is provided in a collaborative way. Social networks provide good samples of various topics of interest in computing environments. By allowing users to create content, social networks are becoming a key issue in research related to the organization and management of large amounts of data, besides being an ideal location for knowledge extraction and application of techniques of data mining environment. However, the huge amount of information does not allow human compilation. It can only be done by an automated reading and selective contents of a particular interest. It represents the so called Internet 2.0, where collaborative content is created. The next evolution is Internet 3.0, where the content will be read and a semantic reasoning will be provided. Concepts such as the semantic web languages for interpretation of its content and the ontologies consolidation applied to the Big Data, configure a new challenge, where the intelligent usage of information available on the Internet can be a way of expanding human knowledge. This work aims to investigate the current situation of dispersed knowledge over the Internet and use it to support strategic planning within the Brazilian public health. It uses only information collected from social networks focused on health. The specific objectives of this work are: (1) to demonstrate the feasibility of using the information available in social networks and the Internet for use in health management; (2) to present extraction methodology based on predefined vocabulary; (3) to establish automatic relevance of data for use in planning decisions in health; (4) to develop a proof of concept to test the proposal.

SOCIAL NETWORKS

The social media environment encourages users to participate and collaborate with new approaches and solutions, criticizing and evolving experiences from their own point of view. Through a timeline and individual variations, it will be possible to develop a range of solutions that meet the vast majority needs. Another aspect is the credibility of social media information. It is directly connect to end-users' approval and acceptance through their own judgment and previous experiences, endorsing or not any assumption or solution presented [1]. Different studies have demonstrated the widespread use of social media like Facebook and LinkedIn for users between 18 and 24 years of age, forty times higher than users above 65 years. Clearly there is a cultural issue in the adoption of technology and a gradual evolution of the percentage in line with the aging population [2]. The incentive for adoption is directly influenced by the ease-to-use operation and immediate results obtained, thus the usability of the tools 2.0 should strengthen aspects of applications, making them more intelligible as possible.

Considering that the content is generated and maintained by users, it is reasonable to consider the contents not true or incorrect in any way. In some situations, the credibility of the information is simply a must, as well as asses its relevance. When thinking about decision-support systems, is desirable to have technological tools which provide different ways to validate and rank information, with emphasis on qualitative data rather than quantitative data, and also be able to create a cross-reference with other data sources. Allowing social media to become a knowledge repository.

There is a very large and good quality volume of information on social media, but the concern is the misinformation and misuse. Inappropriate contents for specific cases and treated as generic content, creating great concern when spread on networks [3]. According to Benvenuto [4], the largest contribution of social media for healthcare is the service networks availability to connected citizens, serving as the main tool for warning, investigation, validation, analysis and interpretation of data, triggering direct action to prevention and reduction of morbidity and mortality.

The capitalization of the opportunity to create an online health community, managed by the government, would change the organizational culture so that the information would not be used only for health surveillance and notifications, but for building and sharing information, rewarding the population through the interconnection between health services and other government agencies [4].

INFORMATION RETRIEVAL

Information retrieval is not limited to texts, but it is applicable to any kind of content. However, the great amount of information is presented as text on medias, such as papers, books, files, web pages [5]. Thus, it is possible to assert that the main interest of a user search, when using information retrieval, is the document content identification. The current technology tries to identify the documents that best resemble the search performed. The validation of the document content itself is still subject of research for greater significance according to the user intentions, and so is the quality classification response.

It is important to understand how the selected documents will produce the necessary result, bringing to the user the knowledge that is required. This situation is divided it into: (1) semantic knowledge, which combines the words and their syntactic structures to conceptual properties; (2) knowledge domain (or context), that adds meaning to the concepts. The ultimate goal is to introduce, by using ontologies, the knowledge that can be semantically associated to questions or queries with the selected documents. Ontology aims to define the representation of something and its definition. Thus, it seeks to understand their relationship and unambiguous features. A set of ontologies is able to promote the understanding and the analysis of a specific domain, organized through their characteristics and relationships. The Internet has promoted a wide variety of graphical user interface languages according to the representation of ontologies. The concept of HTML, and later XML, which make use of tags, or markers, identifying the meaning of the contents, was widely used. Consequently, it allowed the creation of an environment for constructing ontologies, combining the concepts, the usage rules, the relationships, among other features in order to build taxonomies [5].

The main purpose of the usage of ontology is this work is the conceptualization and specification of diabetes mellitus from the perspective of an information retrieval environment, which will allow more efficiently documents search, as well as the organization of search schemas to be performed. The semantic was used to summarize and visualize information in various areas of business, and to what concerns this, in medicine. This technology is directly dependent on a knowledge domain that represents the concepts and semantic relationships between terms for the processing of natural languages, such as the Unified Medical Language System – UMLS [6].

The UMLS codes relationships, and even the relationships themselves, are semantically constructed and prioritized in order to promote greater significance when using between terms in the domain [6]. The application of knowledge in the information retrieval process offers benefits through better search results ascertained. Therefore, the use of ontologies applied to specific areas is recommended. The semantic involved in specific domain is used at all stages of the information retrieval process. Figure 1 represents the simplest retrieving process.

The purpose of introducing ontologies mechanisms for indexing and searching documents, is the identification of ontological similarities, and to prepare an environment which provides a support for retrieving information based on semantics, as illustrated in Figure 2. Studies of information retrieval techniques began in the 1950s, and even today its main concepts are used. The ultimate goal is to present the user the most relevant documents from an ordinary survey. It uses spatial models, probabilistic inference networks and vectorization, in order to optimize processes through semantic significance and context, even if the documents are in different languages or are in different media [4].

The importance of the document selection is directly linked with the completeness of the document description. This complete description, by its turns, depends entirely on the understanding of the document contents so it can be indexed semantically. Therefore, it is necessary to evaluate the relevance of a document with respect to another document submitted.

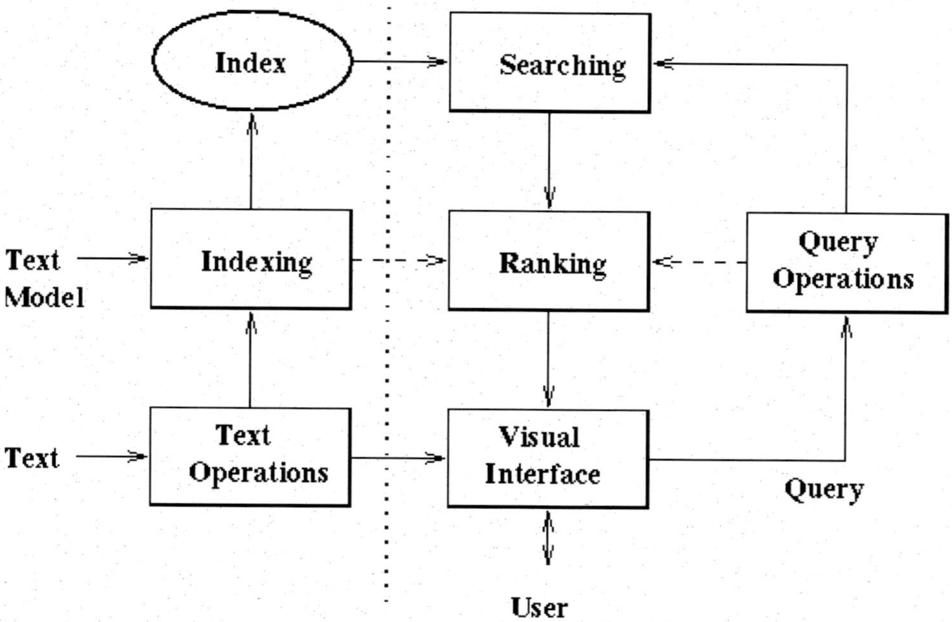

Figure 1. Topological changes over the contour performed by the level-set method.

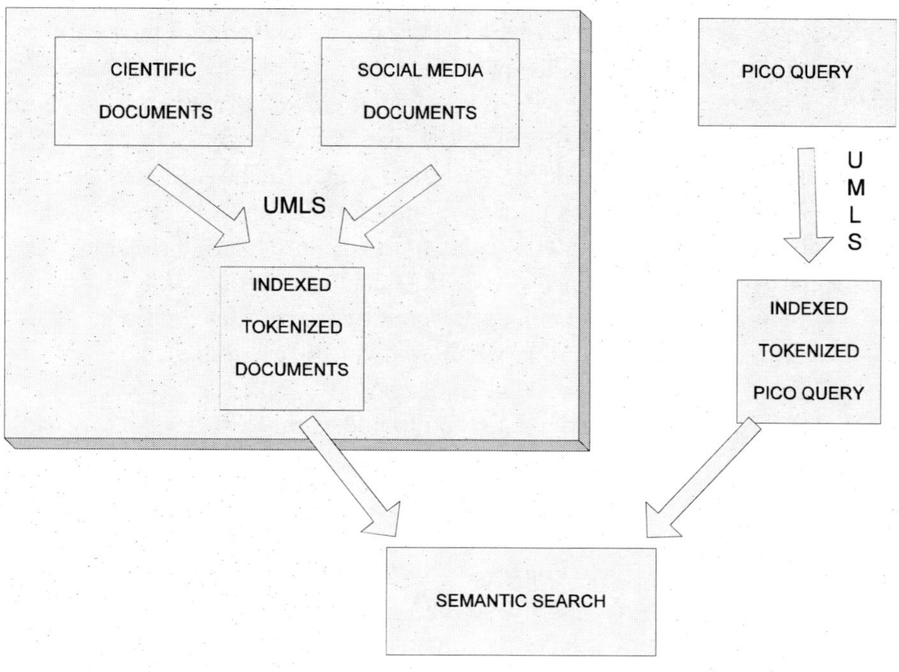

Figure 2. Software basic modules and features.

When using the search on an engine and reading just one of the results obtained, it is questioned the importance of the remaining results to the initial query. Hence, it seems to be interesting a new search based on the similarity between the document read and the next document to be presented. The documents indexing is facilitated by introducing specific vocabulary that supports the context of its document.

The introduction of ontologies also provides greater complexity, since it requires mapping both documents and search questions to the ontologies. Moreover, relations among the documents also allow the establishment of real significance to documents. The method to compare the documents in order to retrieved information for the user query uses features, where several algorithms and approaches are tested. The most common models are [1]: boolean, vectorial and probabilistic.

Natural Language Processing (NLP) is a branch of artificial intelligence and linguistics, which seeks to allow computers to understand what is said in written or oral statements. Considering words as a primitive object, a NLP seek for the relationship between statements and semantic meanings. Thus, it is defined as the use of computational algorithms for processing spoken and written language. The act of extracting fragments of text documents and associating it with the terminology allow the gradual identification of ontologies. Under the clinical context, the UMLS (Unified Medical Language System) provides a set of suitable metadata in medical articles. The use of the Internet 2.0 as an effective source of information for health, guided by evidence-based medicine, will be directly related to the engagement of the users-patients [1].

Public Health and Internet 2.0

The SUS (Sistema Único de Saúde – Unified Health System), a Brazilian state social program, recognizes the universal and egalitarian access to healthcare services and actions, in a hierarchical network. According to law nr. 8080/1990, the National Management of SUS is responsible for drafting and lead the National Strategic Planning with technical cooperation with states, municipalities and the Federal District [7, 8].

By incorporating evaluation as a systematic practice in the various levels of health services, managers can use information for defining intervention strategies. Notice that there is a large amount of information regularly recorded by health services that are not used for the analysis of health status or definitions of priorities and the reorientation of practices. This information is composed by unstructured data. The information flow within the SUS starts at basic healthcare facilities where a primary care software is used, until the data reaches the federal level. Then, the data is compiled and made available for research. The current management model relies on software related to family health, SIAB (Sistema de Informação da Atenção Básica – Primary Attention Information System) strategy [9], recently replaced by the e-Health AB, which comprises several health programs such as the Hypertension and Diabetes Program - Hiperdia.

The term diabetes mellitus (DM) refers to a metabolic disorder heterogeneous etiologies, characterized by hyperglycemia and disturbances in the metabolism of carbohydrates, proteins and fats resulting from defective secretion and/or insulin action. The DM has increased its importance because it is associated with dyslipidemia, arterial hypertension and endothelial dysfunction. It is considered a health condition Primary Attention, that is, a good management of this problem, even in primary care units, prevents many hospitalizations and deaths from cardiovascular and cerebrovascular complications [10].

Social networks can provide a demographic profile of the population, identify locations, groups and so on. A collaborative interaction with the networks allows to understand what the population/network needs, listening to their spontaneous demands. Likewise, once listening to people/network, one can realize how difficult it is to access to health facilities and services.

The evidence-based medicine has become a scientific process, using methodology capable of measuring the results the process or action necessary to obtain them [11]. The use of evidence-based medicine requires an understanding of the following assumptions [12]:

- Use information from systematic, reproducible and unbiased studies, in order to increase confidence in the prognosis of therapeutic effects and usefulness of diagnostic tests;
- Understanding of pathophysiology is necessary but insufficient for clinical practice;
- Understand certain rules of evidence to evaluate and apply effectively the medical literature.

The PICO framework allows the structuring approach to health information in order to deal with the complex content from unstructured documents of any kind, even web pages, facilitating aspects of searching through own vocabularies and application-specific semantics. The (P) Patient or Problem is characterized by the identification of the subject or object that is being evaluated; (I) Intervention is the action considered to be the best option of treatment available at the problem context; (C) Comparison phase is the main alternative to the Intervention which is used as control to evaluate the results of the intervention; and (O) Outcomes presents the possible consequences based on the suggested interventions [13]. Table 1 presents an example of PICO framework applied to the diabetes.

Table 1. PICO methodology applied to the diabetes

Diabetes	
P	People with diabetes type I or II, suffering from foot ulcers of neuropathic, ischemic or neuroisquêmica type. Without restriction as to the presence of infection at the start of the study. Studies that included people without diabetes at baseline were included in the study and studies using other types of ulcers (e.g., venous or vasculitis) were used, since there was separation in the analysis of the results (diabetes vs. no diabetes, no ulcer diabetic ulcer x diabetic)
I	Any topic or healing agent for wounds that contained silver in its composition, used alone or in combination for the treatment of foot ulcers in diabetics. There were no restrictions on works that used antibiotic treatments, equipment for pressure relief or curative side simultaneously
C	The comparison could be with no dressing, dressing placebo (identical, but without silver) and dressings/topical agents without silver in its composition
O	Proportion of ulcers completely healed, the total change in ulcer area, duration until complete healing or change the total area and signs and symptoms of clinical infection.

Health and welfare issues are widely available at Internet, people publish and seek more knowledge on these subjects. Several specific thematic portals and social networks began to aggregate health professionals, patients and institutions, exchanging and collaborating with each other. It provides a rich environment for obtaining information.

Tools based on Internet allow an individual's health to be monitored 24 hours a day, every day. New services, also on the Internet, could be offered, such as a second opinion clinic, emergency monitoring services, data storage and images. Social networks focused on healthcare professionals and patients should support security and quality of information, but it should also provide an approach to offer patients ways of education, prevention, assessment and treatment guidelines. This approach is already underway on platforms such as Sermo (www.sermo.com) and PatientsLikeMe (www.patientslikeme.com) [2].

THE PROPOSED SYSTEM

This project presents a huge number of challenges, such as establishing a way of comparing documents based on free unstructured text, in order to create a set of documents explicitly focused on medicine and another set removed from social networks created by users. Also, it aims to define criteria and relevance to these two sets of documents that demonstrate the presence of health knowledge. The software must perform some basic information retrieval features such as: capture documents from Internet, index the documents, and means for searching documents on this set.

This work also introduce the use of medical vocabulary on indexing step, in order to create a semantic consistence on the documents. Additionally, considering that the purpose of this project is to verify the existence of knowledge on the web, this study use PICO query on the search step, creating a mask of semantic significance. Therefore, to capture documents from Internet, the software implements a well known technology known as web crawler (or spider). This technology consists of navigate through the web sites using the hyperlinks, and download every single page it visits. In order to achieve the goals of this project, we have defined some limits and the scope for retrieving information:

- General diabetes;
- Diabetes in children;
- Diabetes during pregnancy.

This work also defined the initial retrieval web pages that crawlers will be directed to. The healthcare social media was choosen in order to identify users opinion and unique expression of disease evaluated. Generic web pages, including popular social media networks, were used to include ordinary crowd knowledge. Specific medical articles contribute to specialized information.

Therefore, the document corpus was divided into three groups of interest (general diabetes, child with diabetes and pregnant with diabetes) and was obtained from techinical papers (Medline and PubMed), social networks whose main topic is the diabetes (patientslikeme.com and tudiabetes.com), and unrestricted webpages. The distribution of these documents is ilustrated in Table 2.

Table 2. Documents copus description

Source	Group of Interest			Total
	General	Child	Pregnant	
Articles	217	461	172	850
Social Networks	61	48	35	144
Web	243			243

The indexing process is more complex and difficult to implement because it has to handle a lot of documents, tokens and to promote the expected results. Indexing process is also responsible for converting the unstructured document into a semantic structured one using Metamap web service [15]. The index of this process was contructed by using the UMLS [6] entries, and it is storeaged as a UMLS XML file. At this point, the software once again parse this new UMLS XML document, tokenizing its main keys. After that, using UMLS structured vocabulary, the indexing feature identifies the relationships between tokens and further between documents, providing a huge matrix of significance and relevance. The most relevant indexing metrics are calculated and kept waiting for the query input.

A tokenized document table is used in order to map the original document into a semantics structured content based on UMLS. The corpus produced 20.829 unique tokens, and each document have 3.954 token by avearage. Notice that the tokens identification is important, but it is also important to be able to compare each token. Thus, this work uses the token frequency and the inverse token frequency described by Manning et al. [19] to provide this differentiation. Once that all documents are captured and properly indexed, the back-office routines are considered to be completed and the software provide an end-user interface for queries. Understanding the concept of querying using users natural language is a premise, and the objective of validating the methodology of seek knowledge inside ordinary data set. This project proposes the PICO approach, letting the end-user to write freely on the PICO fields. The interface provides filters for origin of information and for disease particularity (general subjects, children, pregnants).

The software query feature, once more, use the semantic conversion from this PICO unstructured query to a UMLS XML file, extract UMLS tokens and use these tokens to fulfill the mission of identify semantic similarities with the original semantic database. The software treat each PICO element individually and then colectively, creating a more representative approach to the query. Hence the query is stored into a so called question-document, wich is divided into other four documents, each one associated to one PICO view. For instance, when submiting 32 queries to the system, it was stored into 128 documents (32x4) and these documents were indexed obtaining the following number of tokens: the P documents have 603 token; the I documents have 306 tokens; the C documents have 281 tokens; and the O documents have 794 tokens. The module of this process are ilustrated in Figure 2.

The semantics search retrieves the documents with better correspondence with the question-documents (query). This correspondence is described by a similarity matrix mapped as a Cartesian product between the query and the documents. This similarity value is obtained by an ordinary distance vector method described at the literature [19], that is:

$$sim(d_1,d_2) = \frac{\vec{v}(d_1).\vec{v}(d_2)}{|\vec{v}(d_1)||\vec{v}(d_2)|} \qquad (1)$$

where $\vec{v}(d_n)$ is the vector representation of the document n.

For instance, consider the following case:

> "CASE 12. Hogarth, a 26 year old botanist, has been diagnosed with depression. Reluctant to take prescribed medication he prefers to try alternative medicines which he feels are better for the body and work just as well. You feel that his disorder would improve more effectively with an SSRI, but he feels strongly that St. John's Wort will be equally as effective."

Where the PICO approach produces:
P = adults with acute shortness of breath presenting to the emergency department.
I = intervention being considered is the BNP and the comparison is the old standby, chest x-ray
C = Pharmacological agents: anti-convulsants, opioids or tricyclic anti-depressants
O = accuracy of the test for diagnosis of congestive heart failure

The semantic search retrieves 1149 documents ordered by their similarity index with the question-document. Considering the top twenty documents, 12 of them are technical articles, 7 documents are obtained from social networks and 1 document is from web content. This arrangement distribution is consistent when other queries are performed. Despite more tests are necessary, it suggests that social network can provide helpful information and that the web content is a tough mining. Another issue obtained the preliminary tests concerns the effectiveness of repository contents. The social networks content represents 11,64% of indexed documents but the queries response have about 39,32% of social networks documents into the top twenty retrieved documents. This suggests either documents obtained from social networks are more significant to user queries, or these documents a better indexed by UMLS.

CONCLUSION

The main purpose of this project is to test Internet crowdsource knowledge existence and its liability when applied to health planning decisions. The development of a software able to retrieve information is not enough to achieve this goal, but it suggests that the information retrieved can be used even if that information is not a technical one, such as popular thoughts. The software itself provides mechanisms to establish the relationship between documents and allows statistics to endorse it.

The initial analysis of software performance and effectiveness consider some different points and issues. At retrieving step, the use of webcrawlers must respect Internet agreements such as allowance in download web pages content according to webmaster/site owner definition. Another issue consists of getting information from "closed" social media networks which only assigned user can access the information posted and also respect users agreement of the web site. From this point of view, the software may have problems getting good information automatically, in special cases, some agreements between researchers and web site companies shall be made specifically for controlled research. More than create indexes on a database, indexing documents for querying requires a lot of experience and different approaches. In this project the indexing process perform more tasks than just attribute weights and relations. The relationships must be consistent with the semantic approach. Thus, just considering documents and tokens frequency and merely attribute weights from it are not enough. In fact the semantic relevance of the terms on the document is evaluated. Therefore, once parsed, the original document is just a reference for further reading. The UMLS XML file is used instead for internal indexing, avoiding the useless set of words and creating the semantic database. Previous works from [16, 17, 18] have suggested that indexing a document with a specific vocabulary must provide better understanding of the document, because semantically it provides the best results, despite of the language used. Another issue considered a limitation, evolves the conversion Metamap web service. This service just use ANSI files, so all retrieved documents despite of their type must be converted to ANSI before parsing. This is supposed to be a simple and automatic task but it may become a problematic if the convertion software leaves some trash behind, that is, not ANSI characters inside the documents.

The query process has to be consistent with the whole software performance. Notice that most of the retrieving and indexing processes are made previously, and that at the time the user starts his query all back-office processes is already done. On the other hand, the parse of PICO query has to be done on the fly, and then process the identification of documents itself. It is also important that the software provides a machine learning using previous queries. Thus, it is possible to train the software previously to its real usage.

The results presentation include a statistic demonstrating the overall of the selection process. It presents percentage of documents by origin, and by specific diabetes subject. It also presents by PICO element the percentage of documents selected. This approach makes the evaluation easier to the user by selecting the document to read it. The most important observations the user must make are to identify the origin of the document and evaluate the different approach of knowledge found. The results obtained so far points to great relevance of social networks knowledge against technical articles and ordinary web content.

The following steps included the increase of the corpus, the development of automation tools for acquiring documents from technical databases, social networks and webpages. It is also necessary to test other similarity indexes and to improve the statitical results about queries response.

ACKNOWLEDGMENT

This research was benefited by the support provided by Coppetec Foundation project Poli-19.257, from Federal University of Rio de Janeiro.

REFERENCES

[1] Metzger, Miriam J., Flanagin, Andrew J. (2011) Using Web 2.0 Technologies to Enhance Evidence-Based Medical Information, *Journal of Health Communication: International Perspectives,* 16:sup1., 45-58, DOI: 10.1080/10810730.2011.589881.

[2] Hesse, Bradford W., Hansen,Derek, Finholt,Thomas, Munson,Sean, Kellogg, Wendy, Thomas, John C., 2010, Social Participation in Health 2.0, Computer (Long Beach Calif). 2010 November; 43(11): 45–52. DOI: 10.1109/MC.2010.326.

[3] Fernandez-Luque, Luis, Karlsen, Randi, Melton, Genevieve B., Health Trust: A Social Network Approach for Retrieving Online Health Videos, (2012) < http://www.ncbi.nlm.nih.gov/pmc/articles/PMC3374533/> Access on November,12, 2013.

[4] Benevenuto, F. (2010). Online Social Networks: acquisition techniques, measuring approaches and future chalenges. In Tópicos em Sistemas Colaborativos, Interativos, Multimidia, Web e Banco de Dados, chapter 2, pages 41–70. Brasilian Society of Computation, Belo Horizonte, Brasil (in portuguese).

[5] Singhal, Amit, Modern Information Retrieval: A Brief Overview, (2001) < http://singhal.info/ieee2001.pdf > Access on December, 8, 2013.

[6] Vieira, Fabíola Sulpino. Avanços e desafios do planejamento no Sistema Único de Saúde. Brasília: Ministério da Saúde. Ciência and Saúde Coletiva, 14(Supl. 1):1565-1577, 2009 (in portuguese).

[7] Kleba, Maria Elisabeth, Krause, Ivete Maroso, Vendruscolo, Carine, O. Planejamento Estratégico Situacional no Ensino da Gestão em Saúde da Família, 2011, Texto Contexto Enferm, Florianópolis, 2011 Jan-Mar; 20(1): 184-93 (in portuguese).

[8] Brasil. Ministério da Saúde. Secretaria de Atenção à Saúde. Departamento de Atenção Básica. Rastreamento/Ministério da Saúde, Secretaria de Atenção à Saúde, Departamento de Atenção Básica. – 1. ed., 1. reimpr. – Brasília: Ministério da Saúde, 2013. 95 p.: il. – (Cadernos de Atenção Primária, n. 29) ISBN 978-85-334-1729-8 (in portuguese).

[9] Brasil. Ministério da Saúde. Secretaria de Atenção à Saúde. Departamento de Atenção Básica. Estratégias para o cuidado da pessoa com doença crônica: diabetes mellitus/Ministério da Saúde, Secretaria de Atenção à Saúde, Departamento de Atenção Básica. – Brasília: Ministério da Saúde, 2013.160 p.: il. (Cadernos de Atenção Básica, n. 36) ISBN 978-85-334-2059-5 (in Portuguese).

[10] Keselman, Alla, Rosemblat,Graciela, Kilicoglu, Halil, Fiszman, Marcelo, Jin, Honglan, Shin, Dongwook, Rindflesch, Thomas C., Adapting Semantic Natural Language Processing Technology to Address Information Overload in Influenza Epidemic Management, 2010, *Journal of American Society of Informatis and Science of Technology*, 2010 December 1; 61(12): doi:10.1002/asi.21414.

[11] Berretta, Isabel Quint, Lacerda, Josimari Telino de, Calvo, Maria Cristina Marino, Modelo de Avaliação da Gestão Municipal para o Planejamento em Saúde, 2011, Cad. Saúde Pública, Rio de Janeiro, 27(11):2143-2154, nov, 2011 (in portuguese).

[12] Atallah, Alvaro Nagib, Castro, Aldemar Araujo, Medicina Baseada em Evidencias: o elo entre a boa ciência e a boa prática clínica, (1997) Access on March, 9, 2014. < http://www.centrocochranedobrasil.org.br/cms/apl/artigos/artigo_520.pdf>.

[13] Boudin, Florian,Shi, Lixin, Nie, Jian-Yun, Improving Medical Information Retrieval with PICO Element Detection, (2010), Access on December, 12, 2013. < http://dl.acm.org/citation.cfm?id=2128355>.

[14] MetaMap – A tool for recognizing UMLS concepts in Text, <http:// metamap.nlm.nih.gov/> Access on August, 20, 2014.

[15] Keselman, Alla, Rosemblat,Graciela, Kilicoglu,Halil, Fiszman, Marcelo, Jin, Honglan, Shin, Dongwook, Rindflesch, Thomas C., Adapting Semantic Natural Language Processing Technology to Address Information Overload in Influenza Epidemic Management, 2010, *Journal of American Society of Informatis and Science of Technology,* 2010 December 1; 61(12): doi:10.1002/asi.21414.

[16] Huang J., Dou D., Dang J., Pardue J. H., Qin X., Huan J., Gerthoffer W. T., Tan M. Knowledge Acquisition, Semantic Text Mining, and Security Risks in Health and Biomedical Informatics. *World J. Biol. Chem.,* 2012; 3(2): 27-33 DOI: http://dx.doi.org/10.4331/wjbc.v3.i2.27.

[17] Styltsvig, Henrik Bulskov, Ontology-based Information Retrieval, 2006, 196p., Thesis (Philosophy) – Faculties of Roskilde University, 2006.

[18] Manning, Christopher D., Raghavan, Prabhakar, Schütze, Hinrich. An Introduction to Information Retrieval. Cambridge, England: Cambridge University Press, 2009. 569p.

In: Models and Methods for Supporting Decision-Making … ISBN: 978-1-63485-173-2
Editors: Carlos N. Bouza, Flávio L. de Mello et al.

Chapter 7

APPLYING FUZZY MODEL TO MAP VULNERABILITY AREAS OF TRYPANOSOMA CRUZI TRANSMISSION

Samanta Cristina das Chagas Xavier[1], Marcello Goulart Teixeira[2], André Luiz Rodrigues Roque[1], Ana Maria Jansen[1] and Luiz Felipe Coutinho Ferreira da Silva[3,*]

[1]Laboratory of Tripanosomatid Biology, Oswaldo Cruz Foundation (IOC/FIOCRUZ), Rio de Janeiro, Brazil
[2]Departament of Computation Science, Mathematics Institute, Federal University of Rio de Janeiro (UFRJ), Brazil
[3]Laboratory of Cartography, Military Institute of Engineering (IME), Rio de Janeiro, Brazil

ABSTRACT

We have developed a novel approach for Chagas disease prediction. We tested the method of spatial fuzzy inference approach as a diagnostic tool of the environmental variables which regulate the *Trypanosoma cruzi* transmission in nature. The set of primary and secondary variables were treated by the fuzzy method of spatial inference in order to build an integrated model. This model demonstrated the possibility to use this novel approach in order to identify areas with different degrees of risk, thus allowing a continuous and integrated representation of the variables involved in the *T. cruzi* transmission in nature. The output data obtained can be used to support decision making in epidemiological surveillance of Chagas disease and are certainly an example that can be applied to several other parasite infections in distinct areas.

Keywords: Chagas disease, *Trypanosoma cruzi*, fuzzy logic

---

* Corresponding author: Luiz Felipe Coutinho Ferreira da Silva. Email: felipe@ime.eb.br.

INTRODUCTION

The observation of nature demand us to admit uncertainty, instability and changeability. That is because we, always have to keep in mind that natural phenomena occur in complex matrices with elements that are completely interdependent [1, 2]. Natural phenomena do not present defined contours or limits and; therefore, are constantly changing. These changes is most of times faster than our theoretical (conceptual or taxonomical) limits in which we insist that these phenomena must fit. This is exemplified by our attempts to define reservoirs, an issue that has been modified over time [3-6]. Communication requires that objects, living things and natural phenomena receive names, are ordered and classified. However, while a classification system allows the exchange of information, experiences and thoughts, this same ordering system can also restrain the advance of a conceptual framework.

Reconciling both the analytical and the holistic approaches is the great and most interesting challenge of studying multi-host parasites, such as *Trypanosoma cruzi*. A complex system similar to this one needs to be studied as a whole because it is impossible to understand the function of such a complex network focusing solely on one part of it. Paradoxically, one must also consider the individual components of the system if aims to understand the whole phenomenon [7].

Actually, each mammalian species constitutes a complex, multivariate and changeable living system, exercising different selective pressures on their parasites in the different environments where they occur. All of the host species select subpopulations of **T. cruzi** in a unique way, and present different infection patterns that depend on numerous macro (landscape) and micro (individual peculiarities) variables [8, 9].

The classical methodology of mapping works with discrete units and sharp boundaries; thus, not considering transition areas. Nevertheless, environmental and biological phenomena are typically continuous and exhibit a gradual transition from one to another characteristic [10, 11]. Unlike the classical methodology, spatial analysis by the fuzzy inference method is able to model the spatial distribution of a continuous biological phenomena, representing its distribution and association in a more realistic way. This modeling can enhance and facilitate decisions [12].

Despite the use of mathematical and computer models is still restricted in the social sciences (mainly due to the low interaction between the areas of knowledge involved) it is observed that the representation of systems and phenomena of the real world through mathematical models is possible, and has shown great advances in recent years [13]. One example is the fuzzy logic developed by Zadeh in the 1960s. The strongly nonlinear nature of the problems, uncertainty and subjectivity is inherent of biological data, although this unpredictability is normally neglected in conventional models. The correct representation of the problems are possible when we make use of appropriate mathematical tools, such as the fuzzy logic.

The modeling by fuzzy logic allows us to incorporate multidisciplinary expert knowledge in the evaluation process. Despite poses a paradigm break in comparison to the valuation methodologies based on classical logic, fuzzy theory facilitates dialogue between the professional of exact sciences, responsible for computational implementation, and experts from different biological areas because it allows the use of linguistic variables and simplistic logical rules. It is worth to emphasize that the participation of a higher number of experts involved in the definition of fuzzy sets (and their evaluation) result in more reliable answers [14]. Such logic has been currently vastly used in biological modeling due to its peculiar features, especially the capacity to model complex and non-linear problems in a simple way.

The introduction of fuzzy sets for dealing with inaccurate concepts was first proposed by Zadeh [15]. The conception of fuzzy logic came up from the perception of Zadeh of the rapid decrease in the quality of information provided by the traditional mathematical models when challenged with increasing system complexity that arises from the way in which the variables of a system are represented.

According to Katinsky [16], fuzzy logic can be defined as the part of mathematical logic dedicated to formalize principles of uncertain or approximate reasoning; therefore, closer to human thinking and natural language. Silva [17] refers to the natural phenomenon, in which, usually, the boundaries between continuous surfaces do not occur brusquely in the majority of cases. Fuzzy logic can perceive a gradual transition is seen from a feature to another, creating ambiguous areas.

In this sense, the theory of fuzzy logic results in a greater refinement of the data modeling, allowing the representation of attributes spatial variation on continuous surfaces. The fuzzy membership specialists make possible the incorporation of knowledge in a quite realistic way, resulting in more coherent scenarios that are less subject to error. The modeling and mapping of a complex and multivariate system resulting from the application of fuzzy inference to the data is expected to reflect the knowledge of the consulted experts [18].

The data modeling approach and mapping employing the theory of fuzzy logic has already been proposed and used in the evaluation of areas at risk of radiation exposure [19], at risk of neonatal death [20], at risk of matrix construction [21], identification of areas at risk of landslides [22] and epidemiological prediction method for dengue outbreaks [23].

This methodology was also used in South Africa, in the river basin of KwaZulu-Natal to identify areas where conditions would favor the occurrence of cholera. An expert system and a fuzzy map of the cholera epidemic in that region were created. Applying this model, it was possible to identify that the subsequent spread of cholera depends primarily on socioeconomic factors [24].

In this context, we described the method of spatial fuzzy inference to implement a model capable to integrates distinct factors that involved with the risk of transmission of *Trypanosoma cruzi,* an primarily wild enzooty parasite, responsible for one of the most important parasitic infections in Americas, the Chagas disease [25, 26]. A prospective model was adopted to define potential risk areas of *T. cruzi* transmission in the municipalities of Belém and Abaetetuba, both from Pará State and the ones that currently display the higher number of acute cases in Brazil [27]. A PhD thesis was concluded, in which we demonstrate for the first time the application of fuzzy inference to map risk areas, supporting the decision-making in epidemiological surveillance of Chagas disease [28].

Thus, a fuzzy model Mamdani type was built using *Fuzzy Logical Toolbox* of MatLab application (R2007b version) [29], which were based on the previously stablished rules to map the Chagas disease risk areas in the Amazon region. The model consisted on a fuzzy network of five layer inferences (Figure 1-5 illustrates the flowchart of the fuzzy hierarchical structure for evaluating the risk of transmission DCA) and 30 inferences (Table 1), which comprised from data of Chagas disease cases, besides mammal, entomological, environmental and meteorological data. Figure 1 shows the variables and inferences made to reach an index related to the disease, similarly Figures 2, 3 and 4 are related to the entomological, mammalian and environmental aspects, respectively. Figure 5 shows the final inference aggregating the different aspects considered. The figures are related to Table 1. Initially, the input data were set in fuzzy values, in terms of linguistic sets (high, medium and low). For each output variable, we created three fuzzy sets (high, medium and low risk). The input and output variables were represented by trapezoidal type functions of relevance defined by a, b, c, and d parameters in the last 4 columns of Table 1. The fuzzy input and rules base Mamdani type were formulated from the knowledge of both consulted experts and data from literature data. The membership functions of fuzzy sets related to these variables in the network have been defined by groups of specialists from each area. Initially the network for inferences was built combining all the possible rules. After this, the rules were presented to the group of experts to validate the decision support of decision from our system, related to the degree of relevance of the variables in fuzzy sets. Thus, the suggested changes were incorporated after each visit. Additionally, a sensitivity evaluation process was performed to identify the contribution of each inference rule output and to detect and remove rules that have not been activated in the system. The model also allowed us to incorporate in the evaluation process the knowledge of experts from the various areas involved in the construction of the rules. The output data was reversed from the fuzzy values though the centroid technique, and normalized at a set interval in accordance with the maximum and minimum values defined by the specialists. After those steps, we performed a sensitivity analysis of the system in which all inferences were tested to evaluate the contribution of each one of the proposed model and to determine the calibration values. The sensitivity analysis showed that the fuzzy model was sensitive to the established form of fuzzy sets, the number of fuzzy sets, the nature of the rules and the employed validation techniques.

The modeling of the system was completed and validated in tests with data from nine localities from the two previous cited municipalities Belém and Abaetetuba. Our results indicated a surface determining different degrees of risk of *T. cruzi* transmission in both areas. The map obtained resulted from the application of fuzzy inference and reflects the knowledge of the consulted experts (Figure 6).

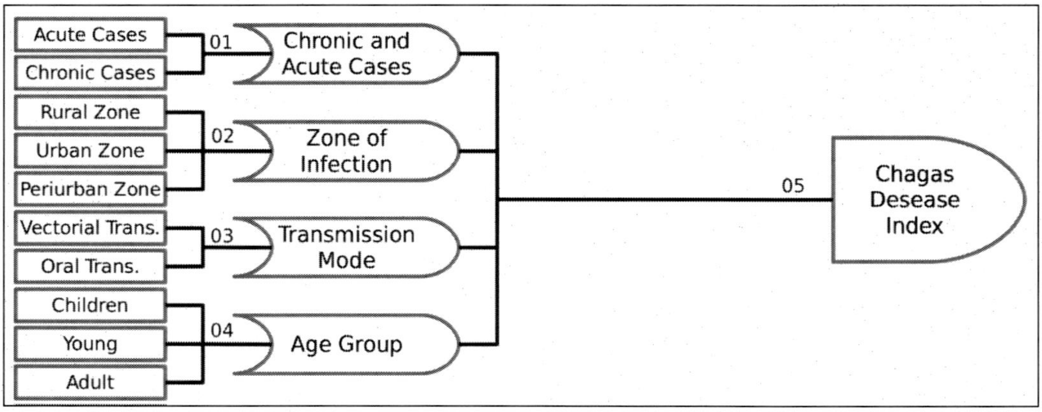

Figure 1. Chagas Disease Index.

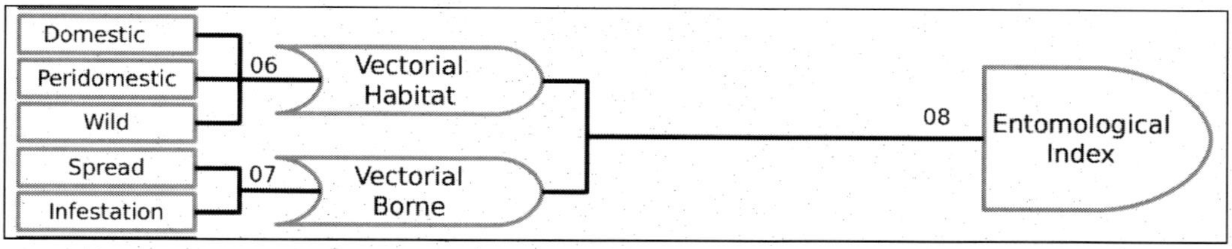

Figure 2. Entomological Index.

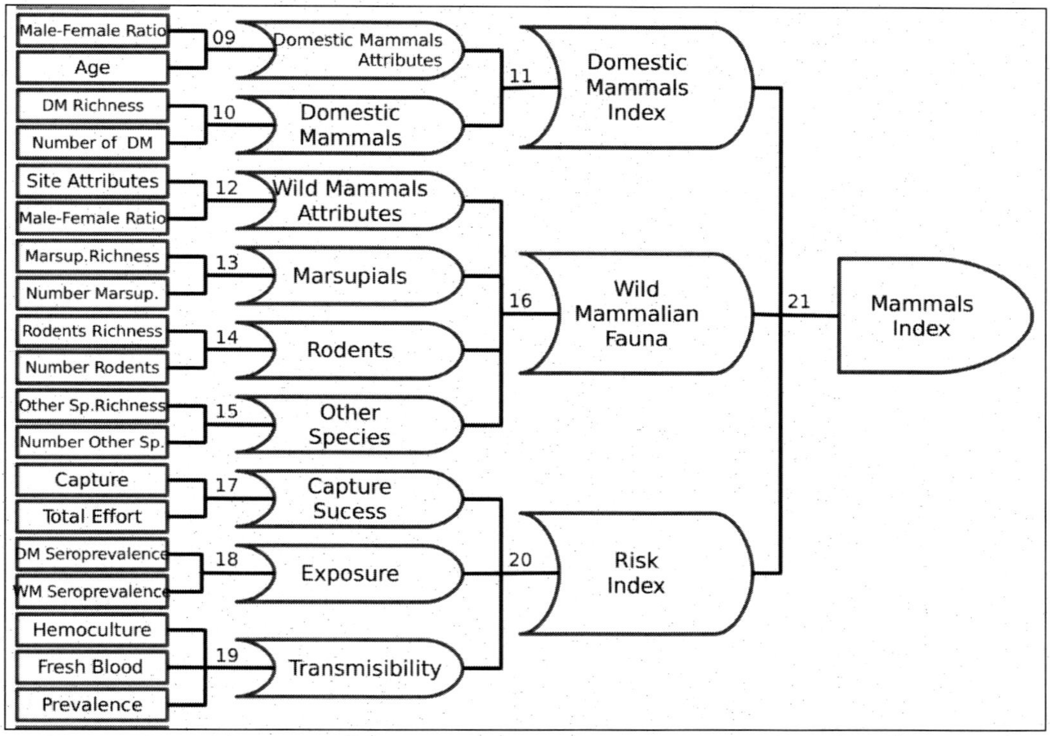

Figure 3. Mammals Index.

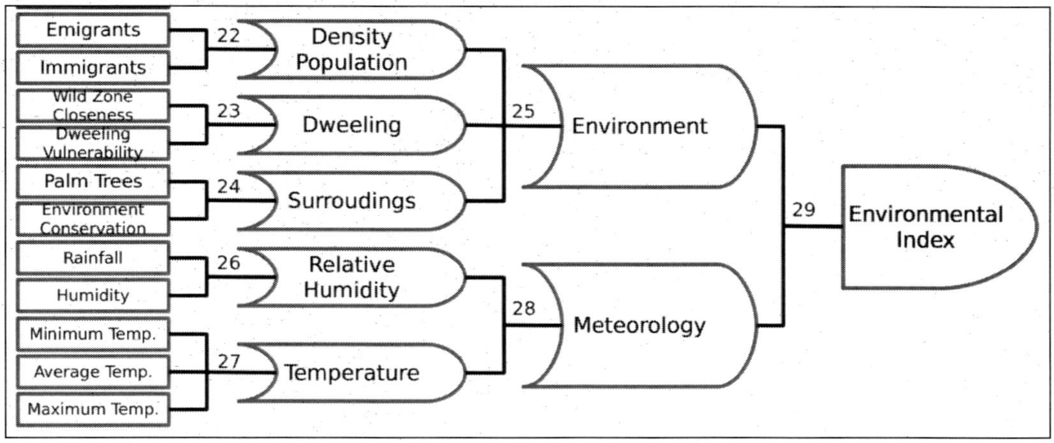

Figure 4. Environmental Index.

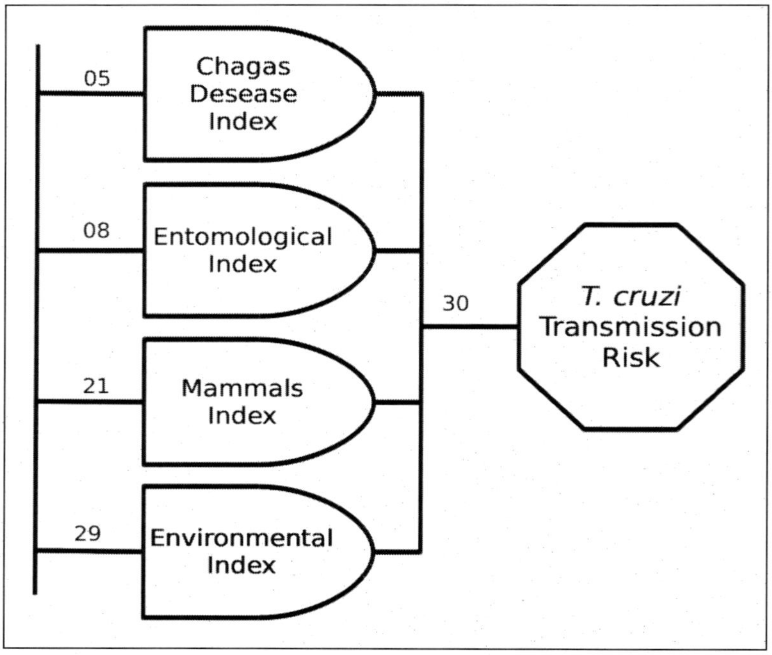

Figure 5. *Trypanosoma cruzi* transmision risk.

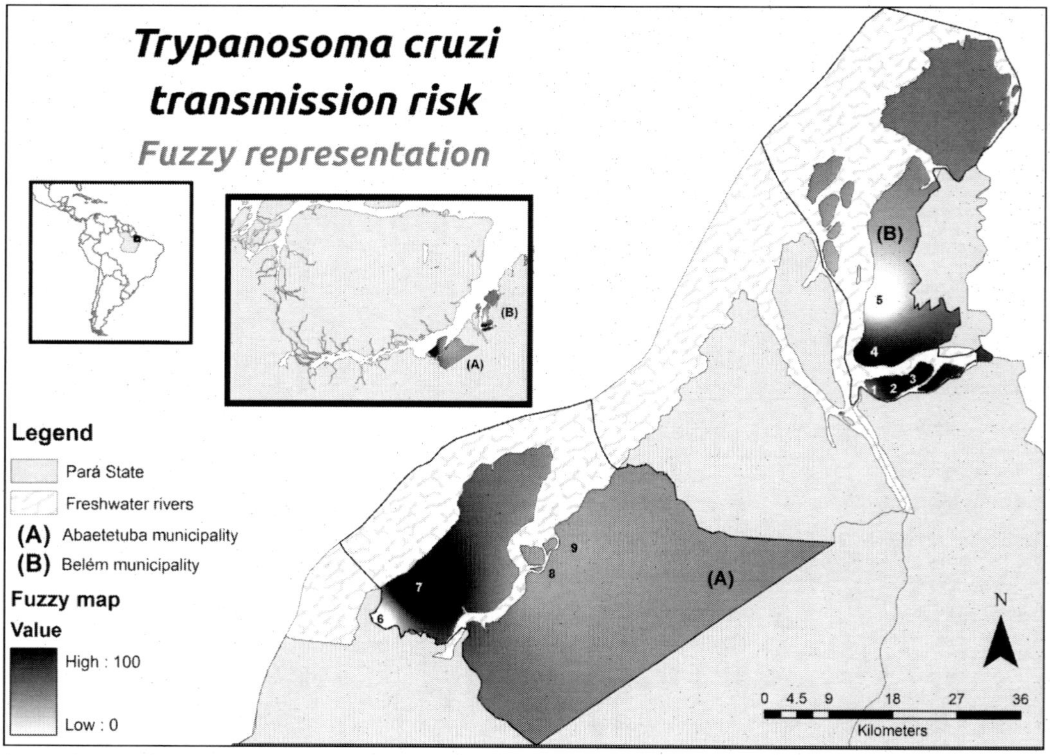

Figure 6. Map of the different degrees of risk of *Trypanosoma cruzi* transmission resulted from the application of fuzzy inference. (A) Abaetetuba municipality (6 - Panacaueira; 7 - Ajuaí; 8 - Genipaúba; 9 - urban area. (B) Belém municipality (in the urban portion: 4 - Jurunas and 5 -Val-de-Cães and on the islands: 1- Pato, 2 – Combu and 3 - Murutucu.

Thus, it was possible to identify regions with higher risk of transmission, which was consistent with the data available in the scientific literature of those localities that are the ones with the highest concentration of case numbers. These areas highlighted by our fuzzy map are the priority ones for epidemiological surveillance in Chagas disease in the state of Pará [30, 27].

CONCLUSION

It was demonstrated that this *T. cruzi* transmission risk model provides the possibility of working with non-probabilistic uncertainty based on the theory of fuzzy sets, allowing the inclusion of non-quantitative variables in the model, reflecting more accurately the reality of the studied areas.

Fuzzy models like this are highly promising for evaluation *T. cruzi* (and potentially all other parasite) transmission risk areas. The resulted fuzzy map represented the occurrence of cases by the graduation of its contours, which is inherent to the fundamentals of fuzzy logic and coherent with the dynamics of a parasite infection. The output data obtained can be used to support decision making in epidemiological surveillance of Chagas disease in these areas and are certainly an example that can be applied to several other parasite infections in distinct areas. The fuzzy map using a *dégradé* color variation is inherent to fuzzy logic fundamentals and coherent with the representation of this kind of problem in decision-making support.

Table 1. Trapezoidal association framework parameters (Membership) of the set of fuzzy functions determined by experts

Hierarchical Fuzzy Decision Tree to TRANSMISSION RISK							
Variable	I/O	Domain	Linguistic terms	a	b	c	d
Inference 1							
Acute Cases	Input	[- 1, 50]	Low	- 1	0	5	10
			Middle	5	10	15	20
			High	15	20	50	50
Chronic Cases	Input	[- 1, 50]	Low	- 1	0	10	13
			Middle	10	13	20	25
			High	20	25	50	50
Chronic and Acute Cases	Output	[- 1, 110]	Low	- 1	0	15	20
			Middle	15	20	40	50
			High	40	50	100	110
Inference 2							
Rural Zone	Input	[- 1, 50]	Low	- 1	0	5	10
			Middle	5	10	15	20
			High	15	20	50	50
Urban Zone	Input	[- 1, 50]	Low	- 1	0	5	10
			Middle	5	10	15	20
			High	15	20	50	50

Table 1. (Continued)

Hierarchical Fuzzy Decision Tree to TRANSMISSION RISK							
Variable	I/O	Domain	Linguistic terms	a	b	c	d
Inference 2							
Periurban Zone	Input	[- 1, 50]	Low	- 1	0	5	10
			Middle	5	10	15	20
			High	15	20	50	50
Zone of Infection	Output	[- 1, 110]	Low	- 1	0	15	20
			Middle	15	20	40	50
			High	40	50	100	110
Inference 3							
Vectorial Transmission	Input	[- 1, 50]	Low	- 1	0	5	10
			Middle	5	10	16	20
			High	16	20	50	50
Oral Transmission	Input	[- 1, 50]	Low	- 1	0	3	10
			Middle	3	10	18	23
			High	18	23	50	50
Transmission mode	Output	[- 1, 110]	Low	- 1	0	15	20
			Middle	15	20	40	50
			High	40	50	100	110
Inference 4							
Children	Input	[- 1, 50]	Low	- 1	0	3	8
			Middle	3	8	15	20
			High	15	20	50	50
Young	Input	[- 1, 50]	Low	- 1	0	5	8
			Middle	5	8	15	20
			High	15	20	50	50
Adult	Input	[- 1, 50]	Low	- 1	0	5	8
			Middle	5	8	15	20
			High	15	20	50	50
Age Group	Output	[- 1, 110]	Low	- 1	0	15	20
			Middle	15	20	40	50
			High	40	50	100	110
Inference 5							
Chronic and Acute Cases		[- 1, 110]	Low	- 1	0	15	20
	Input		Middle	15	20	40	50
	OI-01		High	40	50	100	110
Zone of Infection		[- 1, 110]	Low	- 1	0	15	20
	Input		Middle	15	20	40	50
	OI-02		High	40	50	100	110
Transmission mode		[- 1, 110]	Low	- 1	0	15	20
	Input		Middle	15	20	40	50
	OI-03		High	40	50	100	110

Hierarchical Fuzzy Decision Tree to TRANSMISSION RISK							
Variable	I/O	Domain	Linguistic terms	a	b	c	d
Inference 5							
Age Group		[- 1, 110]	Low	- 1	0	15	20
	Input		Middle	15	20	40	50
	OI-04		High	40	50	100	110
Chagas Disease Index	Output	[- 1, 110]	Low	- 1	0	15	20
			Middle	15	20	40	50
			High	40	50	100	110
Inference 6							
Domestic Vectorial	Input	[- 1, 1]	Eventual	- 1.00	0.00	0.15	0.20
			Frequent	0.15	0.20	0.40	0.50
			Customary	0.40	0.50	1.00	1.00
Peridomestic Vectorial	Input	[- 1, 1]	Eventual	- 1.00	0.00	0.15	0.20
			Frequent	0.15	0.20	0.40	0.50
			Customary	0.40	0.50	1.00	1.00
Wild Vectorial	Input	[- 1, 1]	Eventual	- 1.00	0.00	0.15	0.20
			Frequent	0.15	0.20	0.40	0.50
			Customary	0.40	0.50	1.00	1.00
Vectorial Habitat	Output	[- 1, 110]	Low	- 1	0	15	20
			Middle	15	20	40	50
			High	40	50	100	110
Inference 7							
Vectorial Spread	Input	[- 1, 110]	Low	- 1	0	15	20
			Middle	15	20	40	50
			High	41	51	100	110
Vectorial Infestation	Input	[- 1, 400]	Low	- 1	0	60	100
			Middle	60	100	180	220
			High	180	220	380	400
Vectorial borne	Output	[-1, 110]	Low	- 1	0	15	20
			Middle	15	20	40	50
			High	40	50	100	110
Inference 8							
Vectorial Habitat		[- 1, 110]	Low	- 1	0	15	20
	Input		Middle	15	20	40	50
	OI-06		High	40	50	100	110
Vectorial borne		[- 1, 110]	Low	- 1	0	15	20
	Input		Middle	15	20	40	50
	OI-07		High	40	50	100	110
Entomological Index	Output	[- 1, 110]	Low	- 1	0	15	20
			Middle	15	20	40	50
			High	40	50	100	110
Inference 9							
Male-Female Ratio	Input	[- 1, 110]	Low	- 1	0	10	15
			Middle	10	15	45	50
			High	45	50	110	110

Table 1. (Continued)

Hierarchical Fuzzy Decision Tree to TRANSMISSION RISK							
Variable	I/O	Domain	Linguistic terms	a	b	c	d
Inference 9							
Age	Input	[- 1, 20]	Baby	- 1.0	0.0	0.6	1.0
			Young	0.6	1.0	1.5	2.0
			Adult	1.5	2.0	12.0	12.0
			Elder	8.5	9.0	15.0	20.0
Domestic Mammals Attributes	Output	[- 1, 110]	Low	- 1	0	10	20
			Middle	10	20	40	50
			High	40	50	100	110
Inference 10							
Domestic Mammals Richness	Input	[- 1, 10]	Low	- 1	0	1	2
			Middle	1	2	4	5
			High	4	5	10	10
Number of Domestic Mammals	Input	[- 1, 200]	Low	- 1	0	20	30
			Middle	20	30	50	70
			High	50	70	190	200
Domestic Mammals	Output	[- 1, 110]	Low	- 1	0	12	20
			Middle	12	20	40	50
			High	40	50	100	110
Inference 11							
Domestic Mammals Attributes		[- 1, 110]	Low	- 1	0	10	20
	Input		Middle	10	20	40	50
	OI-09		High	40	50	100	110
Domestic Mammals		[- 1, 110]	Low	- 1	0	12	20
	Input		Middle	12	20	40	50
	OI-10		High	40	50	100	110
Domestic Mammals Index	Output	[- 1, 110]	Low	- 1	0	10	20
			Middle	10	20	40	50
			High	40	50	100	110
Inference 12							
Site Attributes	Input	[- 1, 500]	Not Wild	- 1	0	40	100
			Wild	40	100	500	500
Male-Female Ratio	Input	[- 1, 110]	Low	- 1	0	10	15
			Middle	10	15	35	50
			High	35	50	110	110
Wild Mammals Attributes	Output	[- 1, 110]	Low	- 1	0	10	20
			Middle	10	20	40	50
			High	40	50	100	110
Inference 13							
Marsupials Richness	Input	[- 1, 20]	Low	- 1	0	2	3
			Middle	2	3	4	6
			High	4	6	20	20

Hierarchical Fuzzy Decision Tree to TRANSMISSION RISK							
Variable	I/O	Domain	Linguistic terms	a	b	c	d
Inference 9							
Number of Marsupials	Input	[- 1, 50]	Low	- 1	0	6	10
			Middle	6	10	15	18
			High	15	18	50	50
Marsupials	Output	[- 1, 110]	Low	- 1	0	15	20
			Middle	15	20	40	50
			High	40	50	100	110
Inference 14							
Rodents Richness	Input	[- 1, 10]	Low	- 1	0	2	3
			Middle	2	3	4	5
			High	4	5	10	10
Number of Rodents	Input	[- 1, 30]	Low	- 1	0	5	7
			Middle	5	7	12	15
			High	12	15	30	30
Rodents	Output	[- 1, 110]	Low	- 1	0	15	20
			Middle	15	20	40	50
			High	40	50	100	110
Inference 15							
Other Species Richness	Input	[- 1, 10]	Low	- 1	0	1	2
			Middle	1	2	3	4
			High	3	4	10	10
Number of Other Species	Input	[- 1, 20]	Low	- 1	0	2	3
			Middle	2	3	4	5
			High	4	5	20	20
Other species	Output	[- 1, 110]	Low	- 1	0	15	20
			Middle	15	20	40	50
			High	40	50	100	110
Inference 16							
Wild Mammals Attributes		[- 1, 110]	Low	- 1	0	10	20
	Input		Middle	10	20	40	50
	OI-12		High	40	50	100	110
Marsupials		[- 1, 110]	Low	- 1	0	15	20
	Input		Middle	15	20	40	50
	OI-13		High	40	50	100	110
Rodents		[- 1, 110]	Low	- 1	0	15	20
	Input		Middle	15	20	40	50
	OI-14		High	40	50	100	110
Other species		[- 1, 110]	Low	- 1	0	15	20
	Input		Middle	15	20	40	50
	OI-15		High	40	50	100	110
Wild Mammalian Fauna	Output	[- 1, 110]	Low	- 1	0	15	20
			Middle	15	20	30	35
			High	30	35	100	110

Table 1. (Continued)

Hierarchical Fuzzy Decision Tree to TRANSMISSION RISK							
Variable	I/O	Domain	Linguistic terms	a	b	c	d
Inference 17							
Capture	Input	[- 1, 100]	Low	- 1	0	9	13
			Middle	9	13	23	28
			High	23	28	100	100
Total Effort	Input	[- 1, 2100]	Low	- 1	0	500	600
			Middle	560	650	800	1000
			High	900	950	2100	2100
Capture Success	Output	[- 1, 110]	Low	- 1	0	15	20
			Middle	15	20	40	50
			High	40	50	100	110
Inference 18							
Domestic mammals Seroprevalence	Input	[- 1, 110]	Low	- 1	0	20	22
			Middle	16	21	40	50
			High	41	51	100	110
Wild mammals Seroprevalence	Input	[- 1, 110]	Low	- 1	0	13	20
			Middle	10	20	40	50
			High	40	50	100	110
Exposure	Output	[- 1, 110]	Low	- 1	0	20	25
			Middle	15	20	40	50
			High	40	50	100	110
Inference 19							
Hemoculture	Input	[- 1, 130]	Fast	- 1	0	30	40
			Slow	30	40	130	130
Fresh Blood Examination	Input	[- 1, 110]	Low	- 1	0	15	20
			Middle	15	20	40	50
			High	40	50	100	110
Prevalence	Input	[- 1, 110]	Low	- 1	0	15	20
			Middle	15	20	40	50
			High	40	50	100	110
Transmisibility	Output	[- 1, 110]	Low	- 1	0	20	25
			Middle	20	25	40	50
			High	40	50	100	110
Inference 20							
Capture Success		[- 1, 110]	Low	- 1	0	15	20
	Input		Middle	15	20	40	50
	OI-17		High	40	50	100	110
Exposure		[- 1, 110]	Low	- 1	0	20	25
	Input		Middle	15	20	40	50
	OI-18		High	40	50	100	110
Transmissibility		[- 1, 110]	Low	- 1	0	20	25
	Input		Middle	20	25	40	50
	OI-19		High	40	50	100	110

Hierarchical Fuzzy Decision Tree to TRANSMISSION RISK							
Variable	I/O	Domain	Linguistic terms	a	b	c	d
Inference 20							
Risk Index	Output	[- 1, 110]	Low	- 1	0	23	25
			Middle	18	25	40	50
			High	40	50	100	110
Inference 21							
Domestic Mammals Index	Input OI-11	[- 1, 110]	Low	- 1	0	10	20
			Middle	10	20	40	50
			High	40	50	100	110
Wild Mammalian Fauna	Input OI-16	[- 1, 110]	Low	- 1	0	15	20
			Middle	15	20	30	35
			High	30	35	100	110
Risk Index	Input OI-20	[- 1, 110]	Low	- 1	0	23	25
			Middle	18	25	40	50
			High	40	50	100	110
Mammals Index	Output	[- 1, 110]	Low	- 1	0	23	25
			Middle	18	25	40	50
			High	40	50	100	110
Inference 22							
Emigrant	Input	[- 1, 110]	Small	- 1	0	15	20
			Medium	15	20	40	50
			Large	40	50	100	110
Immigrants	Input	[- 1, 110]	Small	- 1	0	15	20
			Medium	15	20	40	50
			Large	40	50	100	110
Density Population	Output	[- 1, 110]	Low	- 1	0	15	20
			Middle	15	20	40	50
			High	40	50	100	110
Inference 23							
Wild Zone Closeness	Input	[- 1, 500]	Near	- 1	0	55	90
			Middle	55	90	160	200
			Far	155	200	500	500
Dwelling Vulnerability	Input	[- 1, 110]	Low	- 1	0	10	20
			Middle	13	17	40	50
			High	40	50	100	110
Dwelling	Output	[- 1, 110]	Low	- 1	0	10	20
			Middle	10	20	40	50
			High	40	50	110	110
Inference 24							
Palm Trees	Input	[- 1, 110]	Low	- 1	0	14	20
			Middle	13	20	40	50
			High	40	50	100	110
Environment Conservation	Input	[- 1, 110]	Low	- 1	0	15	20
			Middle	14	20	40	50
			High	40	50	100	110

Table 1. (Continued)

Hierarchical Fuzzy Decision Tree to TRANSMISSION RISK							
Variable	I/O	Domain	Linguistic terms	a	b	c	d
Inference 14							
Surroundings	Output	[- 1, 110]	Low	- 1	0	12	20
			Middle	12	20	40	50
			High	40	50	100	110
Inference 25							
Density Population		[- 1, 110]	Low	- 1	0	15	20
	Input		Middle	15	20	40	50
	OI-22		High	40	50	100	110
Dwelling		[- 1, 110]	Low	- 1	0	10	20
	Input		Middle	10	20	40	50
	OI-23		High	40	50	110	110
Surroundings		[- 1, 110]	Low	- 1	0	12	20
	Input		Middle	12	20	40	50
	OI-24		High	40	50	100	110
Environment	Output	[- 1, 110]	Low	- 1	0	15	20
			Middle	15	20	40	50
			High	40	50	100	110
Inference 26							
Rainfall	Input	[- 1, 400]	Low	- 1	0	100	113
			Middle	100	113	184	210
			High	193	200	400	400
Humidity	Input	[- 1, 110]	Low	- 1	0	30	40
			Middle	33	38	56	64
			High	55	65	100	110
Relative Humidity	Output	[- 1, 110]	Low	- 1	0	16	26
			Middle	16	26	45	55
			High	45	55	100	110
Inference 27							
Minimum Temperature	Input	[- 1, 30]	Low	- 1	0	19	21
			Middle	19	21	25	27
			High	25	27	30	30
Average Temperature	Input	[- 1, 31]	Low	- 1	0	20	23
			Middle	20	22	25	27
			High	25	27	31	31
Maximum Temperature	Input	[- 1, 36]	Low	- 1	0	25	27
			Middle	25	27	29	31
			High	29	31	36	36
Temperature	Output	[- 1, 110]	Low	- 1	0	15	25
			Middle	15	20	40	50
			High	40	50	100	110

Hierarchical Fuzzy Decision Tree to TRANSMISSION RISK							
Variable	I/O	Domain	Linguistic terms	a	b	c	d
Inference 28							
Relative Humidity		[- 1, 110]	Low	- 1	0	16	26
	Input		Middle	16	26	45	55
	OI-26		High	45	55	100	110
Temperature		[- 1, 110]	Low	- 1	0	15	25
	Input		Middle	15	20	40	50
	OI-27		High	40	50	100	110
Meteorology	Output	[- 1, 110]	Low	- 1	0	10	20
			Middle	10	20	40	50
			High	40	50	100	110
Inference 29							
Environment		[- 1, 110]	Low	- 1	0	15	20
	Input		Middle	15	20	40	50
	OI-25		High	40	50	100	110
Meteorology		[- 1, 110]	Low	- 1	0	10	20
	Input		Middle	10	20	40	50
	OI-28		High	40	50	100	110
Environmental Index	Output	[- 1, 110]	Not Favorable	- 1	0	15	20
			Favorable	15	20	40	50
			Very Favorable	40	50	100	110
Inference 30							
Chagas Disease Index		[- 1, 110]	Low	- 1	0	15	20
	Input		Middle	15	20	40	50
	OI-05		High	40	50	100	110
Entomological Index		[- 1, 110]	Low	- 1	0	15	20
	Input		Middle	15	20	40	50
	OI-08		High	40	50	100	110
Mammal Index		[- 1, 110]	Low	- 1	0	23	25
	Input		Middle	18	25	40	50
	OI-21		High	40	50	100	110
Environmental Index		[- 1, 110]	Low	- 1	0	15	20
	Input		Middle	15	20	40	50
	OI-29		High	40	50	100	110
T. cruzi transmission risk	Output	[- 1, 110]	Low	- 1	0	22	25
			Middle	18	25	40	50
			High	40	50	100	110

REFERENCES

[1] Mazzocchi and Mazzocchi F. (2012). Complexity and the reductionism-holism debate in systems biology Wiley Interdiscip. *Rev Syst Biol Med*, 4 (5), 413–427.

[2] Montoya, S.L. Pimm, R.V. (2006). Sol Ecological networks and their fragility. *Nature*, 442 (7100), 259–264.

[3] Silva, E.S., Gontijo, C.M., Melo, M.N., (2005). Contribution of molecular techniques to the epidemiology of neotropical Leishmania species. *Trends Parasitol.* 21, 550–552.
[4] Haydon D.T., Cleaveland S., Taylor L.H., Laurenson M.K. (2002). Identifying reservoirs of infection: a conceptual and practical challenge. *Emerg Infect Dis.* 8, 1468–1473.
[5] Barreto MP, Ribeiro RD. (1979). Reservatórios silvestres do *Trypanosoma* (Schizotrypanum) *cruzi,* Chagas 1909 (wild reservoirs of Trypanosoma (S.) cruzi, Chagas 1909). *Rev Inst Adolfo Lutz*, 39: 2536.
[6] Brumpt E (1936). Precis de Parasitologie (Precis the Parasitology). volume, pg 25, 1084 pp.
[7] Jansen A.M., Xavier S.C.C., Roque A.L.R., (2015). The multiple and complex and changeable scenarios of the *Trypanosoma cruzi* transmission cycle in the sylvatic environment. *Acta Tropica In Press*, Accepted Manuscript online 19 July 2015 doi:10. 1016/j.actatropica.2015.07.018.
[8] Dvorak J.A., (1984). The natural heterogeneity of *Trypanosoma cruzi*: biological and medical implications. *J Cell Biochem*, 24, pp. 357–371.
[9] Deane M.P., Lenzi H.L., Jansen A.M. (1984). *Trypanosoma cruzi*: vertebrate and invertebrate cycles in the same mammal host, the opossum *Didelphis marsupialis Mem Inst Oswaldo Cruz*, 79 (4), 513–515.
[10] Xavier S.C.dC., Roque A.L.R., Lima V.dS., Monteiro K.J.L., Otaviano J.C.R., Silva L.F.C.F., Jansen A.M., (2012). Lower Richness of Small Wild Mammal Species and Chagas Disease Risk. *PLoS Negl Trop Dis* 6(5): e1647. doi:10.1371/journal.pntd.0001 647.
[11] Costa, RO., (2007). Representação Cartográfica de Fenômenos com Limites Indeterminados (Phenomena representation Cartographic with Indeterminate Boundaries). Master of Science dissertation on Cartographic Engineering. *Military Institute of Engineering*. 115 pp. 2007.
[12] Burrough P.A., Frank A.U., eds. Geographic Objects with Indeterminate Boundaries. Gisdata II. European Science Foundation. Bristol: Taylor and Francis. 345 p.
[13] Pelli Neto, A., (2004). Avaliação de imóveis urbanos com utilização de sistemas nebulosos (redes neuro-*Fuzzy*) e redes neurais artificiais (urban property valuation with use of fuzzy systems (neuro-fuzzy networks) and artificial neural networks). In: *Congresso Panamericano de Valuación, XXI* (Panamerican Congress of Valuacion, XXI). Cartagena, Colômbia.
[14] Garcia K.C., Teixeira M.G., Alves C.C., Alves R.N., (2007). Concepção de um modelo matemático de avaliação de projetos de responsabilidade social empresarial (RSE) (Designing a mathematical model for evaluating corporate social responsibility projects (CSR)). *Gest. Prod.*, São Carlos, v. 14, n. 3, p. 535-544.
[15] Zadeh, L. A., (1965). Fuzzy Sets. *Information and Control.* United Kingdom, v. 8, p. 338-353.
[16] Katinsky M., (1994). Fuzzy set modelling in Geographical Information Systems. MsC Thesis, University of Wisconsin-Madsin, US.
[17] Silva J.X., (2001). Geoprocessamento para análise Ambiental (GIS for Environmental Analysis). Rio de Janeiro. 228p.
[18] Moreira F.R.S., (2001). Uso e Avaliação de Técnicas de Integração e Análise Espacial de Dados em Pesquisa Mineral Aplicadas ao Planalto de Poços de Caldas (Use and

Integration of Technical Assessment and Spatial Data Analysis in Mineral Research Applied to Planalto Pocos de Caldas). 160 Dissertação (Mestrado em Sensoriamento Remoto) - Instituto Nacional de Pesquisas Espaciais, São José dos Campos - SP.

[19] Vasconcelos W.E., Lira C.A.B.O., Teixeira M.G., (2010). Development of a new fuzzy exposure model. *Progress in Nuclear Energy* 52, 273–277.

[20] Nascimento L.F.C., e Ortega N.R.S., (2002). Fuzzy linguistic model for evaluating the risk of neonatal death Modelo lingüístico fuzzy para estimação do risco de morte neonatal. *Rev Saúde Pública* 36(6):686-92.

[21] Markowski A.S., Mannan M.S., (2008). Fuzzy risk matrix. *Journal of Hazardous Materials* 159: 152-157.

[22] Pradhan B., Lee S., Buchroithner M.F., (2009). Use of geospatial data and fuzzy algebraic operators to landslide-hazard mapping. *Appl Geomat* 1:3–15.

[23] Buczak A.L., Koshute P.T., Babin S.M., Feighner B.H., and Lewis S.H., (2012). A data-driven epidemiological prediction method for dengue outbreaks using local and remote sensing data. *BMC Medical Informatics and Decision Making*, 12:124.

[24] Fleming G., Van Der Merwe M., Mcferren G., (2007). Fuzzy expert systems and GIS for cholera health risk prediction in southern Africa. *Environmental Modelling and Software*, v. 22, p.442-448.

[25] Coura J.R., Viñas P.A., (2010). Chagas disease: a new worldwide challenge. *Nature*. Chagas Disease Outlook. June. S6-S7.

[26] Coura J.R., Junqueira A.C.V., (2012). Risks of endemicity, morbidity and perspectives regarding the control of Chagas disease in the Amazon Region. Risks of endemicity, morbidity and perspectives regarding the control of Chagas disease in the Amazon Region. *Mem Inst Oswaldo Cruz.* 107(2): 145-154.

[27] Xavier S.C.dC., Roque A.L.R., Bilac D., de Araújo V.A.L., Neto S.F.dC., Lorosa E.S., Silva L.F.C.F., Jansen A.M., (2014). Distantiae Transmission of *Trypanosoma cruzi*: A New Epidemiological Feature of Acute Chagas Disease in Brazil. *PLoS Negl Trop Dis* 8(5): e2878. doi:10.1371/journal.pntd.0002878.

[28] Xavier, S.C.C., (2013). Análise espacial como ferramenta para definição de áreas de risco de emergência de surtos de doença de Chagas aguda no estado do Pará/Samanta Cristina das Chagas Xavier (spatial analysis as a tool for defining emergency risk areas of acute Chagas disease outbreaks in the state of Para/Samanta Cristina das Chagas Xavier). – Rio de Janeiro. xii,140 f.: il.; 30 cm. Tese (Doutorado) – Instituto Oswaldo Cruz, Pós-Graduação em Biologia Parasitária, 2013 (Thesis (Ph.D.) - Oswaldo Cruz Institute, Graduate in Parasitic Biology, 2013). Bibliografia: f. 88-107.

[29] Sivanandam, S.N., Sumathi, S., Deepa, S.N., (2007). Introduction to fuzzy logic using MATLAB. *Heidelberg: Springer*, 430 p.

[30] Roque A.L.R., Xavier S.C.C., Gerhardt M., Silva M.F.O., Lima V.S., D'Andrea P.S., Jansen A.M., (2013). *Trypanosoma cruzi* among wild and domestic mammals in different areas of the Abaetetuba municipality (Pará State, Brazil), an endemic Chagas disease transmission area. *Vet Parasitol* 193: 71–77.

In: Models and Methods for Supporting Decision-Making … ISBN: 978-1-63485-173-2
Editors: Carlos N. Bouza, Flávio L. de Mello et al.

Chapter 8

USAGE OF AUTOMATIC THEOREM PROVING IN THE RECOGNITION OF BRAIN EMOTIONS ACTIVATIONS

Flávio Luis de Mello [*] ***and Edilberto Strauss***
Electronic and Computer Engineering Department,
Federal University of Rio de Janeiro, Rio de Janeiro, Brazil

ABSTRACT

The mental operations associated with emotion are different neural mechanisms that correspond to each emotion degrees. It is notorious that science lacks knowledge on the operation of such mechanisms, despite being known that some regions are related to particular emotions. It is usual to enumerate the relationship <mental process, activation region>, while it would be much more interesting if they explain the brain engine aspects. This chapter presents a technique for modeling human brain as a computable object by using theorem proving and digital image processing. A pattern cerebral activation recognizer knowledge base was created from functional magnetic resonance images in order to systemize the cerebral activation human process for a limited set of emotional stimulations.

Keywords: emotional brain activation, machine intelligence, theorem deduction, functional MR images, volumetric images

INTRODUCTION

This work extends previous studies [1, 2] by presenting more specific details on the emotional brain activation computerized recognition system. A wide range of computer

[*] Computer and Electronics Engineering Department DEL/Poli/UFRJ, Federal University of Rio de Janeiro, Centro de Tecnologia, sl.H212B, Ilha do Fundão, Rio de Janeiro, RJ, Brazil, CEP 21949-900. Email: flavioluis.mello@gmail.com.

applications, designed as pattern recognition systems, has been developed in the domain of Medicine. Ghosh-Dastidar and Adeli, for instance, applied heuristic rules and optimum parameter values to electroencephalograms samples in order to increase the computational efficiency and classification accuracy [3]. Garro, Terracina and Ursino used a multi-agent system for supporting the prediction of three-dimensional structure of proteins [4]. Rizzi et al., implemented an automatic microcalcification cluster detection/localization in digital mammograms by employing a wavelet decomposition [5]. Yoshida and Keserci developed a computer-aided diagnosis of lung nodules [6] by adapting an edge-guided active contour based on the wavelet transform.

This chapter aims at improving the understanding of cerebral activation process by an attempt to model human brain as a computable object. Its originality lays on the fact that there are no computational models for mechanical, spatial and temporal brain activation. The widely available models, such as quantitative finite elements models and neural networks, focus on chemical and cellular processes.

Emotion is one of the complex functions human brain is capable of producing, and the neural mechanisms associated with each mental operation are different. It is known that there are relationships between some cerebral regions and emotions, but science lacks knowledge about such mechanism. From this point of view, it is not sufficient to merely enumerate the relation <mental process, activation region>, as it is currently done. It is necessary to elucidate the aspects related to the mechanical functioning.

Functional brain mapping is an ambitious goal which is far to be reached. Under the currently accepted perspective, there are no individual regions responsible for vision, language, or even reason and social behavior. Actually, there are several systems composed of some interconnected cerebral modules, whose dimension may vary from a neuron to a cytological uniform region. Besides, according to its relative position in the system, each cerebral module contributes to different behavior of brain operation, and for this reason, those modules are not permutable. This is a relevant aspect, since what defines the cerebral function contribution to the system operation is not only the structure itself, but also its spatial location in the system.

Brodmann areas form a cerebral mapping system based on a cytological division, which is widely used as spatial determination of neural activity and as a neurosurgery guide [7]. Furthermore, there is also another mapping technique, potentially more precise, based on a coordinate system called Talairach coordinates [8]. Neuroscience employs both approaches for representing the cerebral activation areas over functional magnetic resonance images (fMRI) [9, 10].

METHODOLOGY

Cerebral activation data associated with emotional stimulus, such as repugnance, fear, sadness, happiness and anger, are not widely available since there isn't a solid testing methodology for fRMI exams. Despite the existence of solid neuropsychological protocols for triggering an emotion, the outcome strongly varies from subject to subject. Besides, fRMI exams are still expensive, what makes their use in large scale applications very difficult.

Neuroimaging literature reveals that the processing of emotions, both pleasant and unpleasant, involves sharing several brain structures. However, some of these structures seem to be exclusively required to positive or negative mental states [11]. Phan et al., provided an interesting paper due to the fact that only few studies consider both positive and negative emotional conditions in their experimental design.

In a previous work recently published [1], fMRI images databases and atlases were used as input data. The present chapter, on its turn, assembled twenty right-handed subjects (25 males and 16 females) in order to provide data for the working set. Each subject was submitted to protocols capable of producing states of repugnance, fear, sadness, happiness, and anger. Each protocol was composed of a sequence of images where emotional snapshots were combined with emotionally neutral images. This procedure supplies a control condition since the use of both types of images allows researchers to compare emotional and non-emotional states. It is important to take into consideration that the correctness of the computer system recognition algorithm is not influenced by the type of data acquisition technique used. Therefore, the described protocol allows the algorithm validation.

In accordance with fMRI experiments, it is important to avoid task interference, thus, a passive viewing situation was used. Participants were not given instructions that might have prompted imitation and/or mental imagery of the images shown.

Brain normalization was also an important feature to be taken into account. Once data are generated from different human samples, it was mandatory to apply spatial transformations in order to perform adjustments based on a default brain model. The adopted model was the one proposed by the Montreal Neurological Institute standard coordinate system brain template [12].

Figure 1 schematically illustrates the methodology phases to obtain a computational model recognizer for cerebral activation dynamics submitted to emotional stimulations. Considering the volumetric images obtained from the data collection phase, it was necessary to define Brodmann areas associated with activation. This task was accomplished during the image processing and the coordinate conversion phases. The former was responsible by the activation center calculation, and the latter was dedicated to locate the corresponding Brodmann area. The data codified by Talairach coordinates were processed by the coordinate conversion phase so as to identify the region which inscribes the activation point.

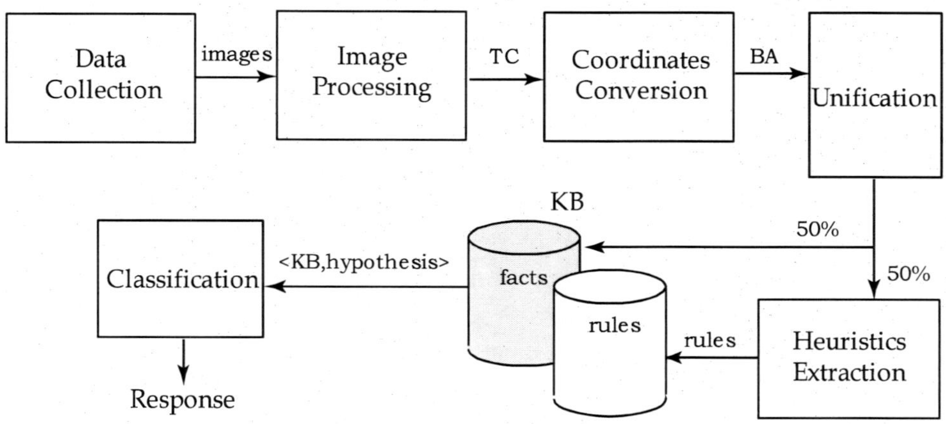

Figure 1. Methodology's block diagram used on the cerebral activation processing.

The Talairach coordinate is defined by a human operator whose expertise subjectively suggests an activation point. If the same human operator had a second chance to indicate the activation point for the identical region, he would probably define a point near the previous coordinate. In fact, one of the disadvantages of using this kind of representation is the absence of a neighboring interval value.

Brodmann areas and volumetric images, on their turn, naturally present an associated error caused by the uncertainty of the neural activation. Therefore, the Brodmann areas labeling was chosen for tagging locations due to its relaxed precision.

The unification phase (Figure 1) corresponds to a data conformation, whose objective was to prepare the obtained data to be represented by logical facts in order to be inserted into a knowledge base (KB). The heuristics extraction was concerned with the search for the identification of production rules that describe the different relationships among the activation volumes during the dynamic cerebral activation process. The number of image frames per test case depends on the medical procedure used to evaluate activation regions. The process described in this paper uses all frames available in image databases, no matter how many of them are provided.

A deterministic finite automaton was used for emotional state recognition. The use of such mechanisms is important since those mechanisms are widely known and accepted as algorithm formalization. Besides, it has at least the same computational power of any electronic device, which allows us to ignore any technological dependency. The identification of such machine, among a sampling space, suggests the existence of a systematic treatment of the problem, that is, it indicates the possibility of constructing a computational model to solve the representation of the brain mechanical activation.

Finally, the classification phase was responsible for identifying an emotional activation sequence. This identification process consisted of performing computational derivation from a hypothesis based on the knowledge described by facts and rules [2]. Hence, if the proposition is proved by the inference machine, it is possible to assert what the corresponding emotional value associated with cerebral activation is.

Coordinates Extraction from Volumetric Images

The main goal of the image processing phase was to define a cerebral activation mathematical center associated with volume activation from a volumetric image. It should be observed that this procedure adds error to the methodology as it generalizes a volume into a mathematical point. However, this error can be minimized since the point was used as a reference to locate the Brodmann volume which encapsulates the punctual activation.

Cerebral function uses several brain regions, which means that one function might use many Brodmann areas at once. Thus, one volumetric image might contain one or more activations simultaneously. The volumetric image was segmented in order to separate all activation volumes. This segmentation was performed by using geodesic snakes [13,14], which guarantees the location of all activation volumes into different bounding boxes.

The original snake implementation [15] uses three energy functionals (see Eq.1). The internal energy controls the tension and elasticity of the curve. The external energy constrains the snake evolution by defining a halting condition according to the gradient difference between the borders and the object exterior. Finally, image energy models the spectral and topological feature variables.

$$E_{snake} = E_{internal} + E_{external} + E_{image} \qquad \text{Eq. (1)}$$

The geodesic snakes represent a geometric approach for image segmentation. It is based on the relation between the original active snake and geodesic calculus (minimum distance curves). It creates a more sophisticated mathematical model, but it also confers a better stability during the contours identification. This kind of approach has been successfully applied to cartographical image segmentation [16,17], which demand much more effort than the fMRI image segmentation discussed in this paper.

Let $C(p):[0,1]\rightarrow R^2$ be a parametric planar curve and $I:[0,a]\times[0,b]\rightarrow R^+$ an ordinary image to be segmented. First, it was defined a function g, dependent of the image gradient ∇I, so that g is strictly decreasing as the image gradient comes closer to regions with high contrast, such as the border of an object in the image. The minimization of the energy equation (Eq.1) is equivalent to minimize Eq.(2), where q is the Euclidean arc length.

$$L_R = \int g(|\nabla I(C)|)\, dq \qquad \text{Eq. (2)}$$

This functional minimization was given by the contour deformation rule of Eq.(3), where k is the curvature and N is the normal unit vector.

$$\frac{\partial C}{\partial t} = (g \cdot k - \nabla g \cdot \vec{N})\vec{N} \qquad \text{Eq. (3)}$$

However, the Eq.(3) just alters the initial curve shape towards the direction of the object border. In order to segment multiple objects inside the image, it was necessary to implement topological changes. These transformations were performed by using Osher and Sethian level-set method [18]. Through this technique, the contour is similar to a level curve, and this curve is one dimension higher than the contour dimension. For instance, the fMRI images are associated with a two-dimensional contour and consequently, it is similar to a tridimensional level curve. This curve is called level-set function and is illustrated on Figure 2.

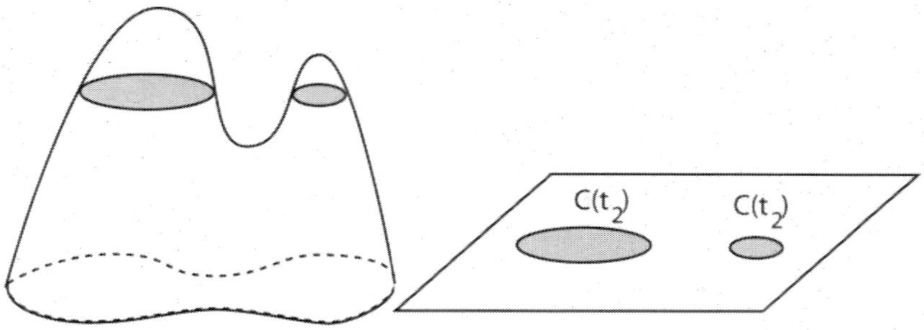

Figure 2. Topological changes over the contour performed by the level-set method.

Thus, by inserting the deformation rule of Eq.(3) into a level-set function, it was possible to obtain the following geodesic active contour of Eq.(4), where Φ represents this tridimensional function.

$$\frac{\partial \Phi}{\partial t} = (g \cdot k - \nabla g \cdot \vec{N})|\nabla \Phi| \qquad \text{Eq. (4)}$$

The analysis of Eq.(4), which defines the geodesic snake, suggests that the $g.\ k$ is analogous to internal energy of Eq.(1) as it controls the contour deformation according to the curvature while it refines its final shape. The $\nabla g.\ N$ provides a similar behavior of the external energy, attracting the curve to the feature border as indicated by the deformation path normal direction. This work uses a function g as described on Eq.(5).

$$g = \frac{1}{1+|\nabla I|} \qquad \text{Eq. (5)}$$

Therefore, at first, it was applied a geodesic snake in order to define the skull's contour line. Then, this line was shrunk and used to initiate another segmentation using the same geodesic snake algorithm. Figure 2 illustrates a volumetric image with eleven activation volumes, being one of these volumes highlighted by its corresponding bounding box.

Once the activation volume is segmented, it was required to compute the activation center. Considering the highlighted volume in Figure 3, one can assert that there is no uniformity in the activation intensity. This phenomenon is indicated by the different gray levels, correctly suggesting that there is an activation gradient on the region of interest. Brighter regions are more active, and thus should contribute more significantly than those less active. This feature is captured by the activation center calculation is given by Eq.(6).

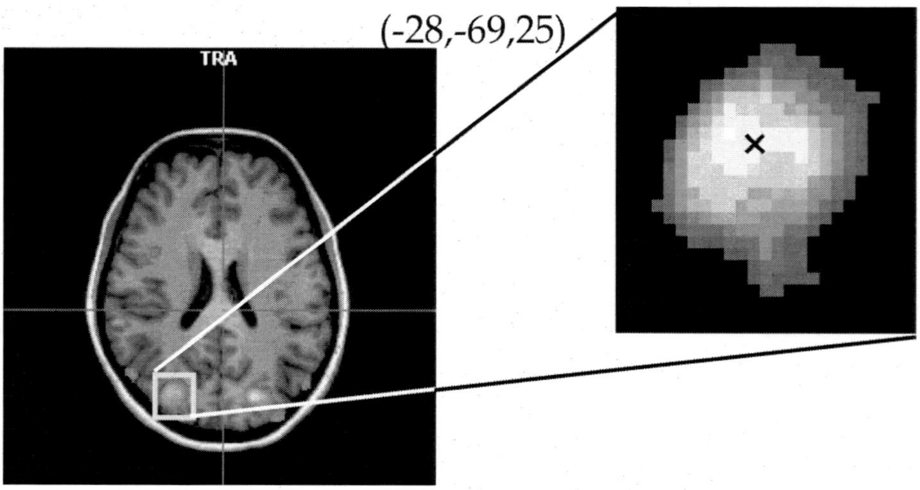

Figure 3. Cerebral activation volume and the determination of a mathematical activation point.

$$P_C = \frac{\sum_i a_i P_i}{\sum_i a_i} \qquad \text{Eq. (6)}$$

The Eq.(6) shows the relative contribution of each activation volume fragment by computing the weighted mean position value for all voxels, and roughly corresponds to the mass center of the region. The value P_i represents the voxel coordinate; ai is the activation intensity; and the coordinate system corresponds to the Talairach System.

Hence, this section explained that the Image Processing phase used geodesic active contours in order to provide image segmentation. It was combined with a ordinary weighted mean position calculus with the purpose of determining the Talairach coordinate associated to the phenomenon.

In this project no filter was applied to the volumetric images. However, it would be interesting to apply the Modified Hartley Transform described by Ahmed [25] because it was conceived for cropping and filtering applications.

COORDINATES CONVERSION INTO VOLUMES OF INTEREST

This stage aims to find the Brodmann volume, which inscribes a coordinate, that is, the activation point. Unfortunately, the authors noticed that there are no computer tridimensional models for human brain divided into Brodmann volumes, which pointed out the necessity of creating such model. During the collection of images to be used on the computational brain model construction, the authors realized that all medical literature references converge to an old book by Sperry et al., [19]. From this reference, three slice images were obtained, scanned, and used to construct vector images. Then, these vector images were spatially transformed in order to be registered over Montreal Neurological Institute default brain surface model [12], which is used by scientific community as a reference model to avoid the brain size variations and deformations.

The Brodmann volumes model was defined by using the planar vector images and a morphing procedure. In Figure 4a, two planar objects (a disk and a star) are used to define the shape from the initial and the final limits of the tridimensional model. Then the morphing procedures produce a tridimensional model where the initial shapes change into the final shape through a seamless transition. For instance, Figure 4b illustrates two slices from Brodmann area 06; the tree dimensional model for this region; and an illustrative overlap between the obtained model and one original slice raster image. The volumes, which compose the brain model, were obtained by using the cross platform suite of computer graphics tools called Blender [20].

Once Brodmann volumes were defined, it was possible to identify the region which inscribes the activation point. This research used a modification of Computer Graphics collision detection [21] routines with the purpose of verifying if the point was located inside of each geometric primitive that compose the three-dimensional model shell.

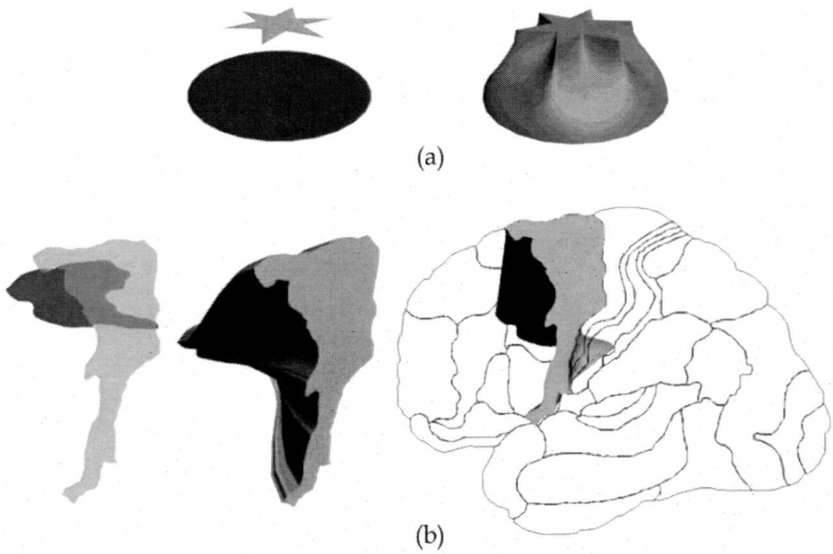

Figure 4. Morphing procedure used to create Brodmann volumes: (a) ordinary morphing shape; (b) BA06 morphing shape.

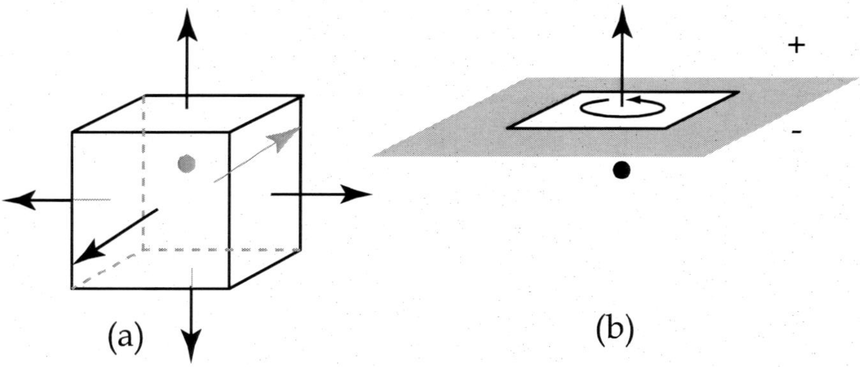

Figure 5. Relative position determination from a point and a given volume: (a) cube with oriented faces and a point of interest inside it; (b) a point in the negative subspace from the top face.

A Brodmann volume was composed of several triangles that together represent the volume shell. For each of these triangles there was a plane containing all triangle vertices. During the construction of the volumes, by using Blender tool, all triangles were counter-clockwise oriented so that their normal vectors were aligned with the outside direction of the volume. As a result, a point inside a volume needs to be located into the negative semi-space of all triangles' planes that define the shell. Figure 5a shows a volume given by an ordinary cube, a point inside this volume, and the oriented faces that constitute the volume shell. Figure 5b illustrates the volume top face, exhibits the orientability, highlights the face plane, and indicates the testing point. Regarding this example, it can be noticed that the point is located on the plane negative semi-space, according to the proposed orientability.

Therefore, the Coordinates Conversion phase allowed cerebral activations to be labeled according to the associated Brodmann volume. These labels were used as input data for the subsequently methodology phases.

KNOWLEDGE BASE CONSTRUCTION

The unification was responsible for preparing all the information obtained through the Broadmann volumes identification stage in order to be represented as propositional facts of a knowledge base (KB). The heuristics extraction corresponds to the production rules determination. Those rules represent the different relation among the activation volumes during the dynamic cerebral activity process.

The emotional states recognition was performed by deterministic finite automata, Turing Machines, represented by finite automata. This kind of approach is quite interesting because those machines are known and accepted as algorithm formalization. Besides, Turing Machines have at least the same computational capacity of any electronic device, which allows avoiding any technological dependency. The identification of such machine proposes the possibility of a systematic treatment to this problem, that is, the feasibility for constructing a computational model capable of solving the brain mechanical activation modeling problem.

In this work, the activation volume was represented by using alpha-numeric symbology. The first two characters of this representation were filled with the same number of the Brodmann volume, which was identified through the Coordinates Conversion phase. The third and last character represented the brain's hemisphere. For instance, the Brodmann volume 23 for the right hemisphere was represented by the symbol 23D. Figure 7 illustrates an automaton associated with modeling of the anger process, beginning at q0 state, where all Brodmann volumes are deactivated. The final states *q7*, *q8* and *q9* signalize that the computation of an emotion has been processed.

The automaton shown in Figure 6 indicates several states arranged into four vertically parallel columns. Each column represents an image acquisition moment when brain activations were captured. The state transition arrows point out the activation/deactivation of Brodmann volumes. The transition between *q1* to *q3*, for instance, suggests that the volume label 10D was no longer activated, and that do volume 11E was activated.

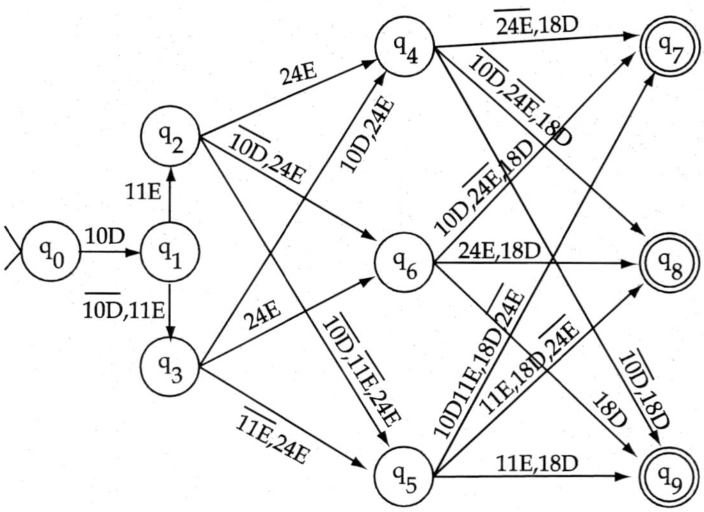

Figure 6. Finite automaton representing the state transition for system recognition associated with anger emotion.

The knowledge base and the inference machine were implemented by using an application called Witty [22, 23, 24], which is a knowledge processing and automatic theorem proving software. The deduction system is refutably complete, which means that if a sentence is a logical consequence of the stored knowledge, then it is possible to infer this sentence by using the system, ignoring the computer limitation of time and storage space.

The knowledge base was divided into two sets: rules and facts. The former contains regulations prescribed by the activation phenomenon for conducting to emotion recognition. The latter were first order logical formulas that represent the information based on real occurrences of a testing exam.

Moreover, considering the transition between *q1* to *q3* in Figure 6, the following rule could be stated:

if state(q1) and not activation(1, 10d) and activation (1, 11e) then state(q3)

This means that if the inference machine state is *q1*, and if the volume 10D was deactivated while the volume 11E was activated, during the second moment of image acquisition, then the inference machine can be changed to the *q3* state.

Table 1. Rules for anger emotion recognition

#	Rule
1	if state(q0) and activation(0,10d) then state(q1)
2	if state(q1) and activation(1,11e) then state(q2)
3	if state(q1) and not activation(1,10d) and activation(1,11e) then state(q3)
4	if state(q2) and activation(2,24e) then state(q4)
5	if state(q2) and not activation(2,10d) and activation(2,24e) then state(q6)
6	if state(q2) and not activation(2,10d) and not activation(2,11e) and activation(2,24e) then state(q5)
7	if state(q3) and activation(2,10d) and activation(2,24e) then state(q4)
8	if state(q3) and activation(2,24e) then state(q6)
9	if state(q3) and not activation(2,11e) and activation(2,24e) then state(q5)
10	if state(q4) and activation(3,18d) and not activation(3,24e) then final(q7)
11	if state(q4) and not activation(3,10d) and not activation(3,24e) and activation(3,18d) then final(q8)
12	if state(q4) and not activation(3,10d) and activation(3,18d) then final(q9)
13	if state(q5) and activation(3,10d) and activation(3,11e) and activation(3,18d) and not activation(3,24e) then final(q7)
14	if state(q5) and activation(3,11e) and activation(3,18d) and not activation(3,24e) then final(q8)
15	if state(q5) and activation(3,11e) and activation(3,18d) then final(q9)
16	if state(q6) and activation(3,10d) and activation(3,18d) and not activation(3,24e) then final(q7)
17	if state(q6) and activation(3,18d) and activation(3,24e) then final(q8)
18	if state(q6) and activation(3,18d) then final(q9)
19	if final(*x) then emotion(anger)

Table 2. Facts for a testing exam

#	Fact
1	state(q0)
2	activation(0,10d)
3	activation(1,11e)
4	not activation(2,10d)
5	activation(2,24e)
6	activation(3,18d)

The anger emotion rules set used in this work did not need so many statements and is listed in Table 1. The process of computing if a certain configuration of Brodmann volumes activation over time represents an emotion, i.e., anger, is equivalent to ask the inference machine if the predicate emotion(anger) can be proved (see Table 1, rule 19). The premise necessary to do so is the existence of any instance of predicate *final(*x)*.

Let Table 2 be the facts describing the activations of a testing exam. The state *q0* is the initial state, where no volume is activated yet; that is, the very moment when the experiment was about to begin. After that, there are succeeding activation and deactivations over four time slots.

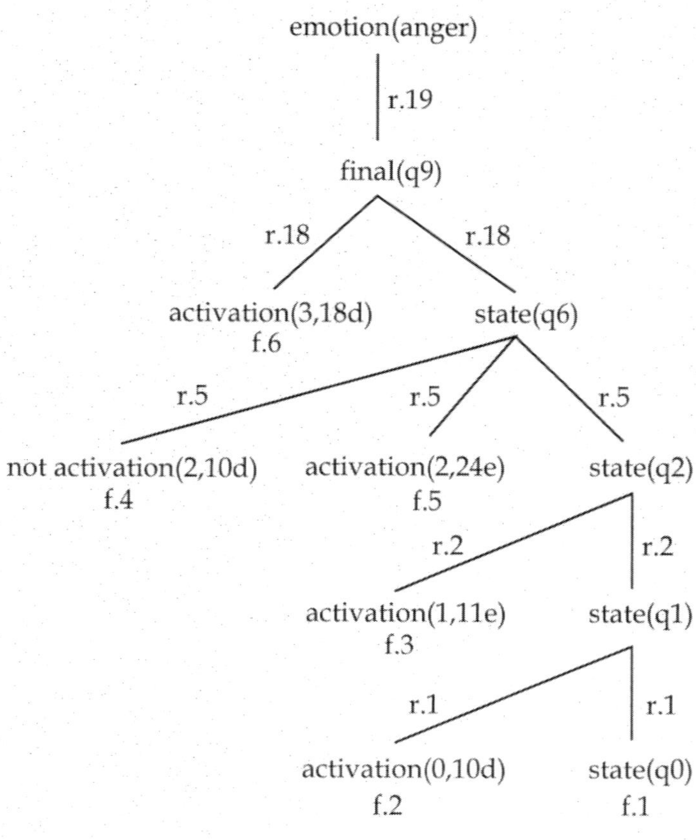

Figure 7. Semantic tree for *emotion(anger)* deduction.

The correct deduction of the predicate emotion (anger) is described by the closed semantic tree in Figure 7. Notice that the deduction was possible only because the computation was able to choose the correct rule composition. In fact, Witty engine provides a backtracking algorithm that allows testing alternative rules to avoid the eventual failure path.

In order to verify which of the five emotions modeled was described by the set of facts from the knowledge base, the proposed methodology triggered five deductions, each one associated with one of the mental states. Note that this kind of approach allowed the recognition of mixed types of emotions, once such combination did exist in the working set.

Besides, as the automatic theorem proving is a straight forward path dependant strategy, it is important to be aware that the knowledge base rules play an important role in deduction algorithm. A successfully proved predicated indicates that a proposition is true over the knowledge base. However, when a predicate is not verified, two situations might have happened: (1) the proposition cannot be proved at all because it is undeductible; (2) the proposition cannot be proved because the knowledge base is incomplete or inappropriate to represent the expertise.

Thus, the construction of the knowledge base described at this section offers the final details for the emotion brain activation recognition. The next section outlines the results obtained through the proposed procedure.

METHODS AND CLASSIFICATION RESULTS

The classification stage identifies the emotional value associated with an emotional activation sequence. This identification process consists of a predicative hypothesis computational derivation according to the knowledge base facts and rules. Therefore, if the proposition is confirmed by the inference machine, it is possible to assert that the emotional activation sequence was identified.

Forty one right-handed normal individuals (twenty five males and sixten females) compose the control and the testing groups of this study, according to the acceptable sample size in medical studies. All subjects stated having no history of neurological or psychiatric disorders. Each of them was submitted to experiments that produced fMRI images for repugnance, fear, sadness, happiness, and anger emotions. Although a twenty sample set is not statistically representative, it can be argued that from the medical point of view it is an appropriate working group.

Table 3. Number of Exams associated to each emotion

Emotion	*Control*	*Testing*	*Successful Recognition*
Anger	20	21	19
Repugnance	20	21	17
Sadness	20	21	15
Hapiness	20	21	18
Fear	20	21	21

Subjects were submitted to an image stream, containing one frame with emotional stimulation and several others emotionally neutral. This routine was adopted as an attempt to provide a control condition in order to produce emotional brain activations isolated from other brain activities.

This protocol is a preliminary sketch and may be reviewed in the future in order to produce better input data. Notwithstanding, correctness is not invalidated since the implemented system do recognize whatever is described by the knowledge bases.

A passive viewing situation was used to prevent the existence of both emotional and non-emotional cerebral activations at the same fMRI image. Moreover, imitation and mental imagery of the images on the part of the participants were avoided by not supplying any kind of instructions during the projection. Immediately after a sequence of images, subjects were asked to indicate what mental state they believe to have been submitted to.

Among all these testing samples, fear emotion recognition reached the highest score. Although this is a good success rate, such value was expected, and even mandatory, since this emotion is described over literature as an easy one to be recognized.

Emotions recognition presented low failure samples; that is, there situations where the proposition could not be deducted by the inference machine. Those failures were similar and occurred because of the insufficient number of exams used during the heuristic extraction phase, which was not able to capture all possible production rules. By increasing the number of exams for composing the control group, thus achieving more samples to define the rules of the knowledge base, it would be possible to reach higher success rate.

Recognition of happiness and sadness states deserves a special attention. The analysis of the deduction failure cases revealed that the knowledge base facts, that is, the testing sample, had no relation with their corresponding rules. Those occurrences were so different from other samples that they could put in question the correctness of the established methods for conducting fMRI acquisition and tagging. The procedures of data collection were reviewed and this doubt was discarded. The unusual occurrences we confirmed as elements from happiness and sadness working sets.

In fact, this demonstrates a naive approach to these mental states. It suggests that the categories of sadness and happiness should have been divided into smaller self-excluded groups, each one representing a different emotion degree. This is a hard task to be accomplished since it is difficult to define what those emotion degrees are. Further studies are needed to provide requirements for such a classification.

Nevertheless, the implemented methodology for emotional brain activation recognition was able to correctly classify 85,71% of all experimental samples. This value of successful classification can be considered a good result.

CONCLUSION

This chapter demonstrated how image processing, computer graphics and theory of computation can be useful on emotion recognition. It was shown a pattern cerebral activation recognizer Turing Machine, derived from functional magnetic resonance images, in order to systemize the cerebral activation human process for a limited set of emotional stimulations. It was explained how to locate volumes of interest over a computational model by using volumetric images as input data. The image segmentation used geodesic snakes with the purpose of extracting multiple activated brain volumes. Then, those volumes were reduced to a mathematical activation point to facilitate the subsequent phases. Moreover, it was described how the computational brain reference model was obtained from ordinary raster images. Besides, this paper explained how to label the mathematical activation point according to its associated Brodmann volume.

Finally, it was shown the usage of an automatic theorem prover, supported by knowledge bases, in order to arrange an fMRI image set according to five categories of emotions. The construction of such knowledge bases has also been presented. The analysis of the recognition results suggests that the five emotion categories considered should be split into more classes. Sadness and happiness groups seem to demand a subdivision, where each subgroup represents a different emotion degree.

The volumetric data image acquisition used only right-handed subjects since left-handed subjects would introduce an additional problem variable. However, it can be speculated, and reasonably accepted, that the presented methodology does provide correct results since a representative knowledge base is constructed. Automatic theorem proving is not concerned with the nature of what is represented by the knowledge base, such as a heterogeneous group of left-handed and right-handed subjects. It just requires an accurate description of the representative features of that collection.

The mathematical activation point is an artificial trick to simplify the identification of the corresponding Brodmann volume. In spite of that, it is interesting to carry out a direct test between the activation volume and the Broadmann volume. The geodesic snakes already provide segmentation through a vector shape. The several shapes from the volumetric image can be used to produce a geometrical model by combining computer graphics tessellation routines.

In addition, it would be ambitious to model not only primary emotions, but also the secondary ones. However, secondary emotions are not innate, cultural dependant, and for this reason, more difficult to be controlled by a medical protocol.

In future works, it is intended to increase the number of exams used on the heuristic extraction stage with the purpose of enlarging its representability. This enlargement requires a revision of the fMRI images acquisition in order to produce better quality input data. Furthermore, the usage of additional fMRI data from databases and atlases will be evaluated. In addition, it would be interesting to classify images using neural networks such as the one proposed by Ghosh-Dastidar and Adeli [26,27]. Moreover, an hybrid Dezert-Smarandache model might be used for pattern recognition such as the one designed by Dahabiah et al.,[28].

ACKNOWLEDGMENTS

This research was benefited by the support provided by Coppetec Foundation, through project Poli-19.257, from Federal University of Rio de Janeiro.

REFERENCES

[1] Mello, F. L; Oliveira, A. A. F.; Strauss, E. "Emotional Brain Activation Model Based on Computer Theory and Digital Image Processing." *17th International Conference on Systems, Signals and Image Processing, pp.*219-222, 2010.

[2] Mello, F. L; Strauss, E. "Machine Intelligence and RMf Image Processing Applied to the Recognition of Brain Emotion Activations." *I Workshop Models and Methodologies to Support Decisions Applied to Health and Environment Management,* Fortaleza/Aracati, 2014.

[3] Samanwoy Ghosh-Dastidar and Hojjat Adeli, Improved spiking neural networks for EEG classification and epilepsy and seizure detection, *Integrated Computer-Aided Engineering 14*, pp. 187-212, 2007.

[4] Alfredo Garro, Giorgio Terracina, Domenico Ursino, A multi-agent system for supporting the prediction of protein structures, *Integrated Computer-Aided Engineering* 14, pp. 259-280, 2007.

[5] Maria Rizzi, Matteo D'Aloia, Beniamino Castagnolo, Computer aided detection of microcalcifications in digital mammograms adopting a wavelet decomposition, *Integrated Computer-Aided Engineering* 16, pp. 91-103, 2009.

[6] Hiroyuki Yoshida, Bilgin Keserci, Bayesian wavelet snake for computer-aided diagnosis of lung nodules, *Integrated Computer-Aided Engineering* 7, pp. 253-269, 2000.

[7] Douglas, R.J., Kevan A. C.M., "Neocortex," In: *The Synaptic Organization of the Brain,* Eds.: C.M. Shepherd, New York: Oxford University Press, pp.389-438, 1990.

[8] Talairach, J., Tournoux, P., *Co-Planar Stereotaxic Atlas of the Human Brain,* New York: Thieme Medical, 1998.

[9] Duong, T., Yacoub, E., Adriany, G., "High-Resolution, Spin-Echo Bold, ad CBF fMRI at 4 and 7 T," *Magnetic Resonance in Medicine,* v. 48, pp.589-593, 2002.

[10] Logothetis, N., Merkle, H., Augath, M., *"Ultra High-Resolution fMRI in Monkeys with Implanted RF Coils,"* Neuron, v. 35, pp.227-242, 2002.

[11] Phan, K.L., Wager, T., Taylor, S.F., Liberzon, I. Functional neuroanatomy of emotion: a meta-analysis of emotion activation studies in PET and fMRI. *NeuroImage* 16, pp.331–348, 2002.

[12] V.S. Fonov, A.C. Evans, R.C. McKinstry, C.R. Almli and D.L. Collins. Unbiased nonlinear average age-appropriate brain templates from birth to adulthood. *NeuroImage,* 47, Supplement 1: 102, 2009.

[13] Terzopoulos, D.; McInernet, T., "T-Snakes: Topological Adaptative Snakes," *Medical Image Analisys.* v.4, pp73-91, 2000.

[14] Caselles, V., Kimmel, R., Sapiro, G., "Geodesic Active Contours." *Procedures of International Conference in Computer Vision Boston,* EUA, p.694–699, june 1995.

[15] Kass, M., Witkin, A., Terzopoulos, D. "Snakes: Active Contour Models," *International Journal of Computer Vision,* pp.321-331, 1988.

[16] Pereira, Cassius Marcelus Ferreira; Mello, Flávio Luis de; Vergara, Oscar Ricardo. "Segmentação de Imagens de Satélite Através de Contornos Ativos Geodésicos." In: *Congresso Brasileiro de Cadastro Técnico Multifinalitário,* 2006, Florianópolis. Proceedings do COBRAC 2006, v. 8, 2006. (in portuguese).

[17] Costa, F. A. L.; Mello, Flávio Luis de; Vergara, Oscar Ricardo. "Contornos Ativos Geodésicos: um Método Alternativo para Sebmentação de Imagens de Satélite." In: Simpósio Brasileiro de Sensoriamento Remoto, 2007, Florianópolis. Anais do XIII Simpósio Brasileiro de Sensoriamento Remoto. *São José dos Campos: Instituto Nacional de Pesquisas Espaciais,* pp. 6027-6033., 2007. (in portuguese).

[18] Osher, S. J. e Sethian, J. A., "Fronts propagating with curvature dependent speed: Algorithms based on Hamilton-Jacobi formulations," *Journal of Computational Physics,* vol. 79, pp. 12–49, 1988.

[19] Sperry, R. W., Gazzaniga, M. S., Boegen, J. E., Handbook of clinical neurology, v. 4, chapter Interhemispherec relations. *The neocortical commissures;* syndromes of their disconnection, Amsterdam, North-Holland, pp. 273–290, 1979.

[20] Blender Foundation, "Blender 2.41," www.blender.org, accessed on november 2008, 2008.

[21] Bergen, G. V. D., *"Collision Detection in Interactive 3D Environments,"* c.4, Elsevier, 2004.

[22] Oliveira, C. M. G. M. Labelled Theorem Proving For Substructural Logics. In: 12th Brazilian Symposium on Artificial Intelligence - SBIA 95, 1995, Campinas. *Lecture Notes in Artificial Intelligence.* Berlin: Springer-Verlag, v. 991. pp. 79-91, 1995.

[23] Oliveira, C. M. G. M. "An Architecture for Labelled Theorem Proving," PhD Thesis, Imperial College of Science, *Technology and Medicine, ICSTM*, 1995.

[24] Witty Inteligência Artificial Ltda., *"Witty – Automatic Theorem Prover,"* www.wittyia.com.br, accessed on april 2010, 2006. (in portuguese).

[25] Ahmed, A.M.T., "Enhanced Frequency Pattern of the 2-D Hartley Transform for a New Crop-Resilient Image Transform," *Integrated Computer-Aided Engineering, 17*:1, pp. 15-28, 2010.

[26] Ghosh-Dastidar, S. and Adeli, H., "Spiking Neural Networks," *International Journal of Neural Systems,* 19:4, pp. 295-308, 2009.

[27] Ghosh-Dastidar S. and Adeli, H., "A New Supervised Learning Algorithm for Multiple Spiking Neural Networks with Application in Epilepsy and Seizure Detection," *Neural Networks,* Vol. 22, pp. 1419-1431, 2009.

[28] A. Dahabiah, J. Puentes, B. Solaiman, "Fusion of possibilistic sources for pattern recognition," *Integrated Computer-Aided Engineering,* 17:2, pp. 117-130, 2010.

In: Models and Methods for Supporting Decision-Making … ISBN: 978-1-63485-173-2
Editors: Carlos N. Bouza, Flávio L. de Mello et al.

Chapter 9

RADIOLOGY INFORMATION SYSTEM WITH KNOWLEDGE REASONING

Sérgio Ricardo Pereira Soares[1,*], Edilberto Strauss[2] and Flávio Luis de Mello[2]

[1]State University of Ceará and Federal Institute of Ceará, CE, Brazil
[2]Electronic and Computer Engineering Department,
Federal University of Rio de Janeiro, Rio de Janeiro, Brazil

ABSTRACT

The purpose of this article is to define an Information System which uses medical radiologic cases in DICOM format in order to create a knowledge repository and an approach to retrieval of the correct cases using keywords. This repository aims to improve the medical radiologists' capacity to provide more accurate and faster diagnoses by using case based reasoning techniques. Besides, it also helps teaching radiological techniques to newly radiologists. The construction of such repository demands to join together various radiologic cases of Magnetic Resonance Image and Computer Tomography equipments, and allows pointing out semantic problems associated to the filling information by the time exams are made. It also suggests that is necessary to create a fulfillment policy of form fields so that later searches can be executed easily and interactively.

Keywords: radiology information system, picture archiving and communication system, digital imaging and communications in medicine, DCM4CHE, case based reasoning

* State University of Ceará, Av. Dr. Silas Munguba, 1700 - Campus do Itaperi, Fortaleza, CE, Brazil. Email: srpsoares@tonanet.com.

INTRODUCTION

The ability to generate and collect medical data in recent years, has undergone an incredible increase with the new technologies that were created. In radiology, it was common to have X-Ray devices generating only 3 or 4 images for each patient. Today we have modern equipment like the Computed Tomography (CT) and the Magnetic Resonance Imaging (MRI), which can generate 2000 images on a survey of only one part of a patient's body.

Several techniques are being developed to improve the handling of the data in this area. In the early 1970s, artificial intelligence (AI) techniques were used to generate knowledge through statistical data on diseases. In the 1980s, these efforts have evolved to CBR [1] techniques (Case Based Reasoning), with the intention to use the knowledge acquired in the previous disease reports to diagnose the current pathology. Today, the information retrieval is the common approach.

This article aims to define how to build an information system (IS) that can provide a retrospective search over a repository of radiological reports, and therefore help the radiologist in his work routine. This proposed system shall be integrated into the existing image system of either a clinic, or a hospital. Once implemented this integration, the system will provide details of previous reports to the radiologist who will be able to use them in order to support his own diagnosis.

HOSPITAL INFORMATION TECHNOLOGY ENVIRONMENT

To understand the process of data collection employed in the information system dedicated to radiologists, it is mandatory perceive the operation of hospitals and clinics, as well as existing sectors and finally how each information system communicates with each other. The sectors of a hospital generate an abundant amount of data, suggesting the need to classify them in order to define their importance in each sector of the hospital environment IT. Is possible to classify the data in three groups:

a) Administrative Data - Existing in any large company and is well known in industrial and service sectors.
b) Financial Data - It have the same characteristics of theadministrative data and are well known in business environments.
c) Clinical Data - These data are private to the medical sector and little studied to date. They can be formed by information from different sectors in a hospital, and also they may be concentrated in a information system known as electronic medical records.

Figure 1 shows the most common sectors of a hospital as well as the information systems communication protocols used, such as DICOM [2] and HL7 [3]. The shaded area defines the sectors that provide clinical data for physicians. The most important sector for the IS in question is the RIS [4] (Radiology Information System), where is located the PACS [5] (Picture Archiving and Communication System). The PACS stores the images and reports in DICOM format.

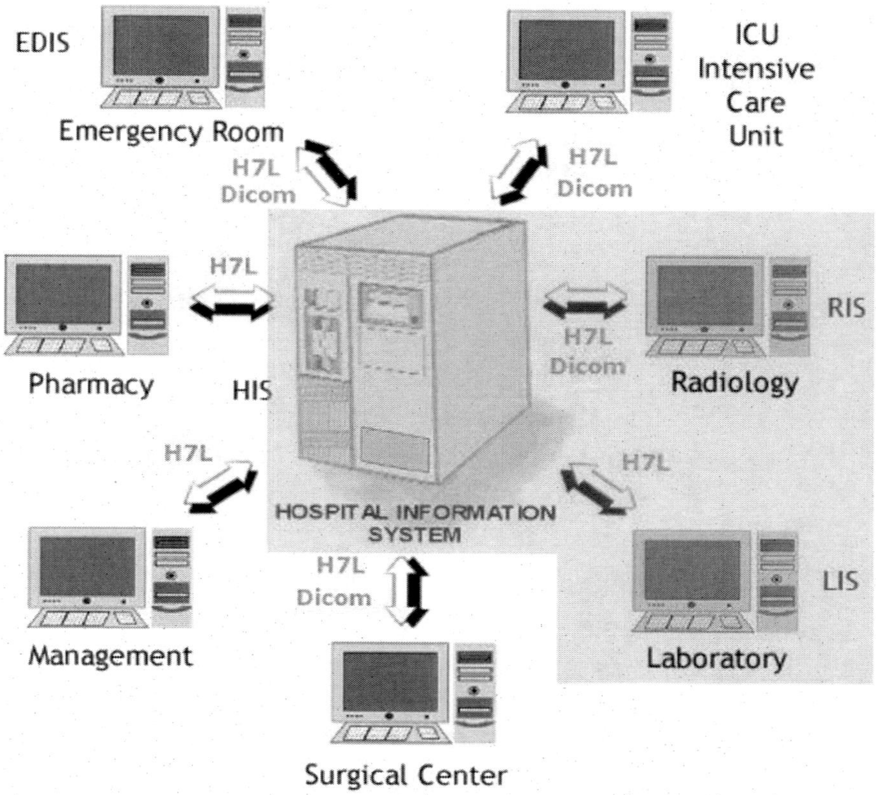

Figure 1. Sectors and protocols used to exchange information.

INFORMATION SYSTEM

This Information System proposal was designed after the dialogue with several radiologists over the hypothetical construction of a radiological cases database. At first, the conceived IS would consist only of reports generated by physicians and stored in text format. However, all interviewee were very categorical that the stored report would be quite useless in future cases analysis, without the images. Therefore, the concept of IS underwent a significant change in its original design, since it would support the storage of images as well.

To implement the proposed IS, it was chosen an open source solution with DICOM protocol support so as to allow storage of the report, i.e., texts and images. In this case, the challenge was the search and the conversion of data in DICOM format, to an easier way of recovering the cases using keywords. The solution was a set of DICOM tools that first makes a search for primary parameters in the database and then converts the reports found to XML [6] format to allow the user to select each case found. In order to build this decision support system, it was necessary to divide the problem into two parts. The first part builds the repository that accepts images in DICOM format and, if necessary, can generate medical reports to be stored. The system can receive the reports of a patient together with the images in DICOM format or can generate and store them in the correspondent patient in the same format.

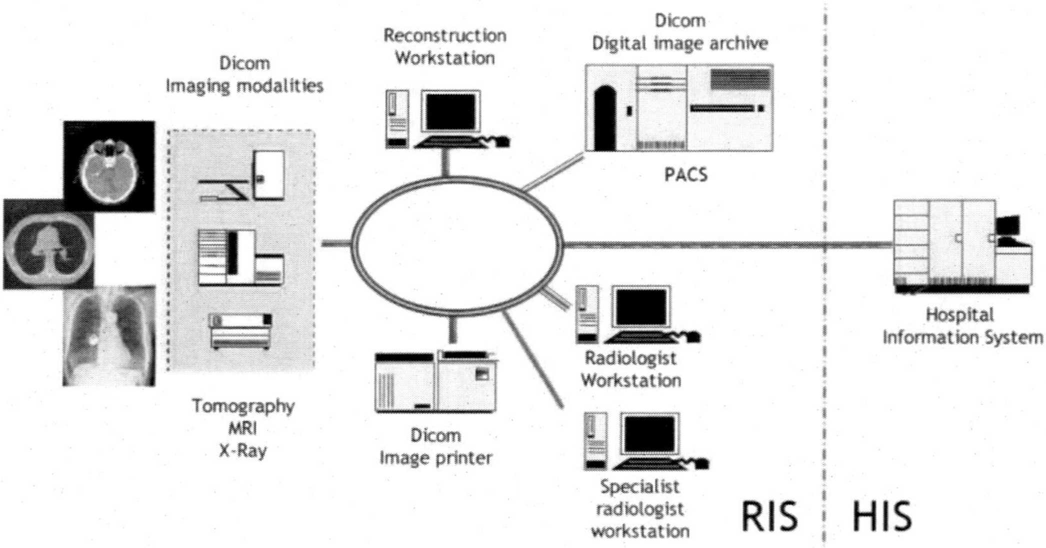

Figure 2. RIS with the specialist medical report station.

The second part is formed by the search engine that makes the recovery of stored cases, according to keywords provided by the physician who is querying the system. Figure 2 presents a detailed overview of the RIS (Radiological Information System) sector, and how the proposed Information System will be connected to the existing infrastructure.

The RIS sector provides the following basic functions for radiologists:

a) Patient registration and exam appointments
b) Patient document control, such as medical claim and previous examinations.
c) Integrated scanner to digitize documents of patients
d) Control clinical reports
e) Report the findings in the exam and provide electronic signatures
f) The possibility to send the report by fax or email to the requesting doctor or patient

The PACS (Picture Archiving and Communication System) is responsible to store and manage images from digital modalities. He often has film scanners so that analogic modalities can be integrated. The basic functions are to reduce the film printing and provide images remotely to doctors or patients (PACS web).

The digital modalities are formed by the devices that generate the images of the patients and are available mainly in the systems listed below:

a) Digital X-ray
b) Computed Tomography CT
c) Magnetic Ressoance Imagers MRI
d) Digital mammography
e) Nuclear Medicine
f) Positron Emission tomography PET

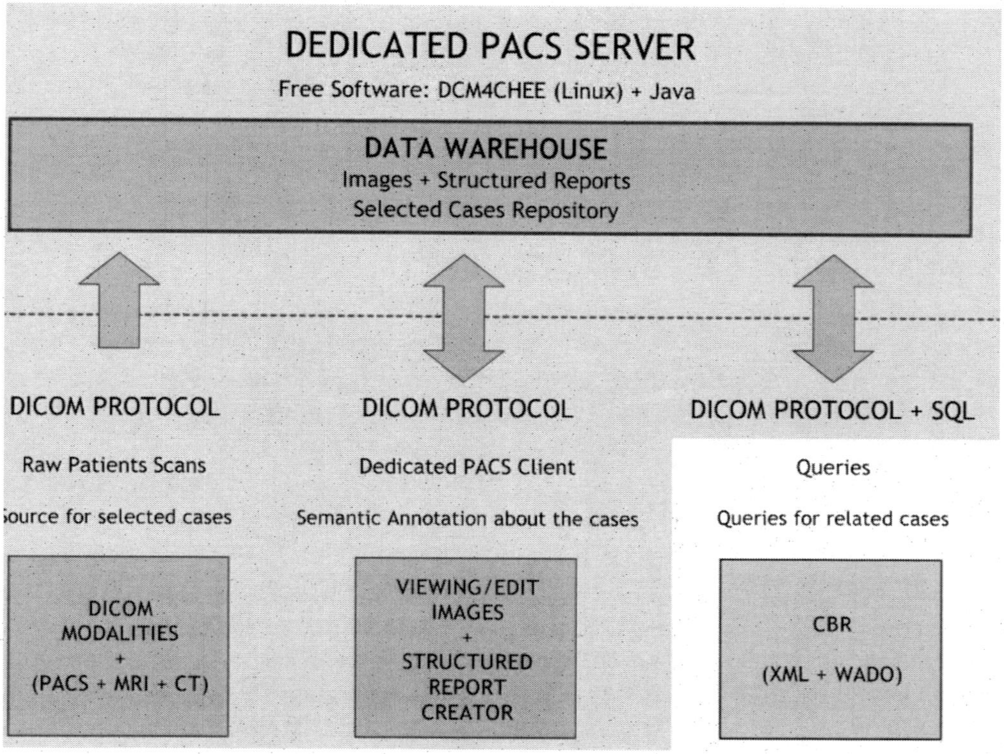

Figure 3. RIS with the specialist medical report station.

The RIS also communicates with the HIS (Hospital Information System) that controls the administrative portion and the financial management of clinics and hospitals. It usually integrates the CIS (Clinical Information System) which implements the electronic patient record among other functions.

The proposed system is able to deal with full cases. They are stored by radiologists by sending images and the structured report [7] to the DICOM server. It consists of programs with the open source GPL [8] standard. The final system is described at Figure 3.

The PACS server uses a dedicated computer with Linux operating system [9] and the database management system MySQL [10]. The utilitarian software DCM4CHEE [11] provides the services compatible to DICOM protocol used in medical services. The use of this protocol was necessary to facilitate the data input on the server without any conversion of the images previously stored in other servers. The radiological images are provided by the modalities or through another PACS server on site. Thus, we can separate the structure of the proposed IS into two parts defined as follows:

a) Dedicated PACS server (DCM4CHE) that stores the images and reports in DICOM format and the Turyon DCM4CHE Lite Viewer [12] software, which offers the option of viewing images and making the report in DICOM, known as structured report. Hence, it is possible to define this system part as the module responsible for collecting the complete cases and loading them into the repository.
b) Set of tools available in DCM4CHE package that supports the cases retrieval using keywords. These tools also converts retrieved DICOM cases to XML format,

facilitating an advanced search. It is also possible to retrieve those cases using SQL [13] commands, some kind of direct access the DCM4CHE database. However, it is suggested to use a tool developed for the DCM4CHE that accesses the database using the framework support. Each option has its difficulties and will be detailed at the following section. This part can be defined as the recovery cases module.

Module to Store Cases in DICOM Format

A dedicated PACS client was used by a radiologist to provide semantic annotation on the cases and to insert the keywords that will be used by the search program later in a query. This search program is based on another open source software called Turyon DCM4CHE Lite Viewer which allows images visualization and structured reports creation.

Figure 4 illustrates the modules of the Turyon software, with the purpose of improving their operation understanding. In a computer server with DCM4CHE PACS installed, the Turyon software establishes a service to provide access from anywhere on the Internet. Yet is also possible to use a VPN (Virtual Private Network) [14] connection, if this service is available. It provides greater security in software connection and data exchange.

The physician connects the client software to the server using a login and a password that are registered in Turyon server. He may have access to certain examinations or even all of them, depending on what have been configured in his user profile. After connecting, the physician will get a screen where all patients will be available so it can generate the report. If no patient is available, is necessary to check if there is a connection to the PACS server. If he gets a connection error message, the connectivity parameters should be checked.

The next step is to select the desired patient to view correlated images and generate the report using the reporting functionality. This function enables the data filling for the report of this patient, which will be recorded in the structured report format, along with the images. This facilitates an easy case recovery by the second part of the program.

The fields available for filling in the report are configured in a way that the physician can inform what was required, what he found when he made the patient exam and what is the conclusion about what was found. Then the report is sent to be stored on a dedicated PACS, along with images of this patient. Only some physicians will have access to enter cases in the database and this have to be defined by the head of the radiology department.

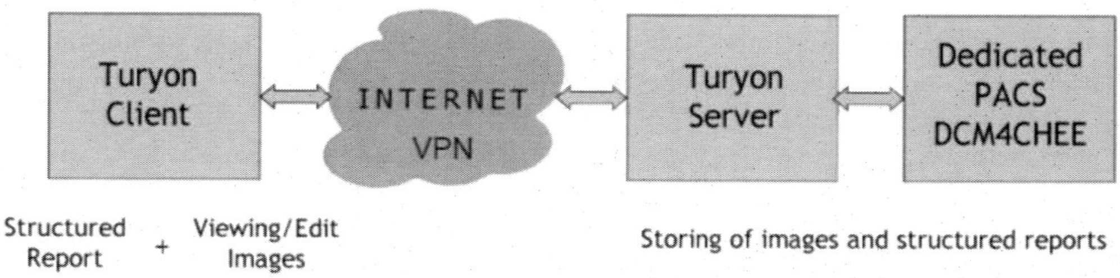

Figure 4. IS diagram for collecting cases.

Recovery Cases Module

The recovery module should start checking the structure of the database to determine which fields should be searched. This structure was not defined here because is very complex and contain several fields that will not be used (detailed information can be obtained at DCM4CHE Database Schema Diagram [15]). Information retrieval can be obtained using three different methods to search:

a) The recovery can be made directly by accessing the DCM4CHE database using the SQL command Full-Text Search (FTS) [16] in the field that store the data structured report. After recovering the data, it will be transformed into a hypertext page using the XML language. This method is risky because if the SQL command is done in the wrong way, it can change the database and damage it. Furthermore, he is not obeying the DICOM standard, which can hinder any other operation, e.g., the display of images.
b) The recovery can be made using the JPDBI [17] DCM4CHE tool available in the framework. It accesses the database using SQL commands, but not directly, which can avoid any damage to the cases already stored. Using the extended query option is possible to search keywords on the field that stores the structured report and the tool will return the patients found. With this list of patients, it is possible to use another command available in the DCM4CHE framework dcm2xml [18] to generate the pages that will be consulted by the physician. The links generated will use the WADO [19] protocol to visualize the images of the selected cases.
c) The recovery can be made using the part of the anatomy of the body selected by the physician with the program dcmqr [20] available in the DCM4CHE framework and then converting the retrieved cases to XML using the dcm2xml command. In this format is possible to make the search of the keywords in the report and eliminate cases that do not have the desired characteristics. The links generated by XML after selection will use the WADO protocol for displaying pictures of the selected case. In this sense, it was chosen the third method of data recovery because it makes all operations without using commands that directly access the DCM4CHE framework database. This approach decreases the risk of corrupting the stored information. However, this method has a problem, it depends on the correct completion of the data when the scan on the patient is performed.

RESULTS ANALYSIS

The first part of the IS was completed successfully and the database was populated with 363 exams from eight different magnetic resonance imagers (MRI) equipments and one computer tomography imager (CT) from more than one manufacturer. This heterogeneous infrastructure is important because it reflex the common resources available in hospitals and clinics. The results were obtained by searching the repository generated, highlighted that the expected fields fill pattern was not strictly obeyed, spoiling the information retrieval of cases. As a practical example, it was made a search in the DICOM field "Study Description" for

Knee examinations (Joelho in Brazilian Portuguese language) and the query result didn't recovered any scans available in the repository. This happened because none of the exams have the "study description" field filled with "JOELHO." This clearly demonstrates that each clinic or hospital provide the database attribute filling according to their own will, which complicates the recovery of semantic instances. Therefore, a fill pattern of examinations must be adopted for every exam in order to resolve this kind of problem.

A query with the word "RM JOELHO ESQUERDO" using the field "study description" provided some relevant results to the query, since was used the semantics defined by the user. A query with the word "JOELHO*" in the field "study description" requests the search program to search for the word KNEE, including patients that have some extra information after the word defined. The query result listed all examinations starting with the word JOELHO and all the others that have the word JOELHO in the beginning of the field and some other information after. However, those queries do not list the patients that have the description "RM JOELHO," once again demonstrating the importance of standardizing the correct completion of the exams.

A detailed description of the queries made in the repository and the results can be found in Soares [21]. As an illustration to the standardization problem of the "study description" field, in Table 1, there are some examples of the different definitions found in the repository for the same type of patient scan in MRI.

Table 1. Some examples of the different definitions for the same type of patient scan for the field "study description"

Type of scan performed	Semantics found
Cervical Spine	CERVICAL
(Coluna Cervical)	COL CERVICAL
	RMCOLUNA CERVICAL
Lumbar Spine	COL LOMBAR
(Coluna Lombar)	COL. LOMBAR
	CRANIO ROTINA^ROTINA
	CRANIO^Brain Dot Engine
Head	CRANIO^ROTINA
(Crânio)	CRANIO
	RM CRANIO
	RM DE CRANIO
	JOELHO DIREITO
	JOELHO ESQUERDO
Knee	MUSCULO ESQUELETICO^JOELHO
(Joelho)	RM JOELHO DIREITO
	RM JOELHO ESQUERDO
Angiogram of the Head	CRANIO ANGIO^CRANIO
(Angio de crânio)	ANGIO^CRANIO
	VASCULAR^ANGIO CRANIO

Table 2. SNOMED DICOM Microglossary code (SDM)

ABDOMEN	ARM	ANKLE	BREAST	CHEST
CLAVICLE	COCCYX	CSPINE	ELBOW	EXTREMITY
FOOT	HAND	HEAD	HEART	HIP
JAW	KNEE	LEG	LSPINE	NECK
PELVIS	SHOULDER	SKULL	SSPINE	TSPINE

Table 3. Codes found in the repository for the field Body Part Examined

ABDOMEN	CERVIX	HEAD	HEART	KNEE
LSPINE	PELVIS			

In order to try to circumvent this semantic problem another DICOM field was selected "Body Part Examined." This DICOM Tag defines the region of the body where the image was generated and have default values defined by the SNOMED DICOM Microglossary (SDM) codes [22] listed in Table 2. These values were used in another DICOM tag called Anatomic Region Sequence that is now deprecated.

In 2007 the DICOM consortium defined a new list of default codes listed in the DICOM document CP 722 – Add cross-reference between Body Part Examined and Anatomic Region [23]. This list contains 112 values and they used the 25 default values from SNOMED.

Checking the completion codes of the DICOM field Body Part Examined in the repository, it was verified that not all images had identification and in most of the exams, this field was empty. The results found are listed in Table 3.

In some exams the problems in this field were even worse, a head exam had all images identified as Heart and other head exam had all images identified as abdomen. Finally another problem was found in several exams, some series have the correct identification while others not. In other to try to identify why this happened it was made a research with the radiology technicians of this equipment and the result for the misidentification of the head exams was very simple. The radiology technician of one of the systems told that sometimes they take protocols from one region of the body to scan another part of the body, because they do not have the correct protocol programmed to use. It was the case of the head exam identified as heart, the head protocol was not programmed in the system and the radiological technician had to use the heart protocols. Using this information, a research on one of magnetic resonance image equipment was made and it the results found were various errors in the programming protocols on this equipment, justifying the results found in the repository. Using this findings, is clear that the first step to implement this IS would be to talk to the radiological technician and ask them to correct the protocols in the system. Not only because of this system, but because it is violating the DICOM rules and could be a problem for other IS in the hospital.

In order to improve the quality of the proposed IS is possible to implement the Case Based Reasoning method described by Aamodt and Plaza [1] to manage and recover the cases in the repository. On the diagram of Figure 5 is possible to verify how the cycle is organized and how it works. The method is initially described by a four cycle process that can provide a continuous updating of cases and the increase of knowledge:

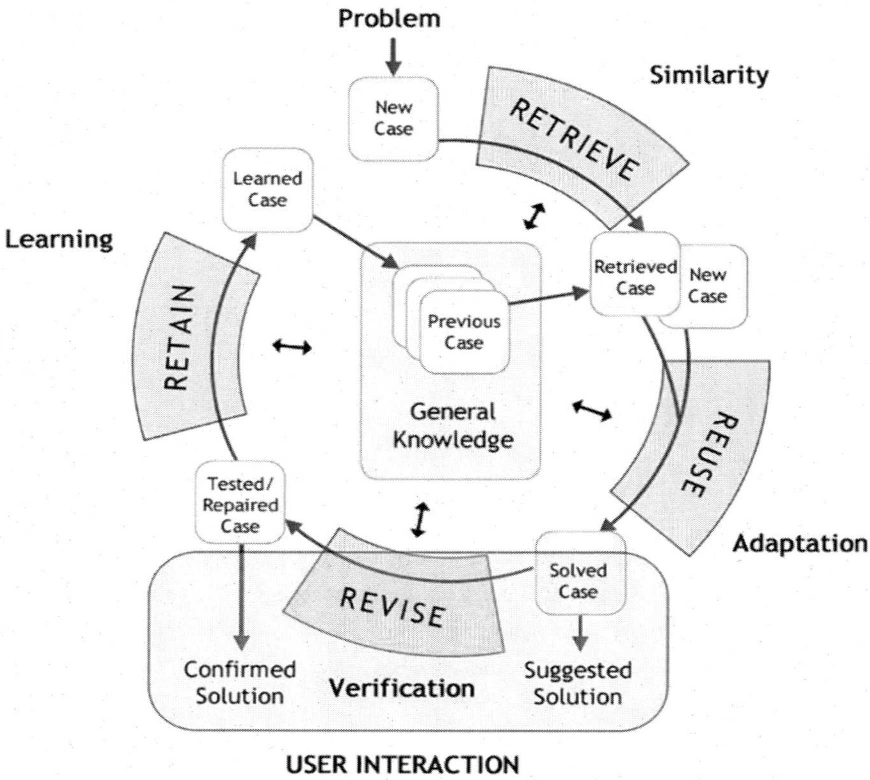

Source: A. Aamodt, E. Plaza [1].

Figure 5. CBR cycle.

a) Retrieve: Using the characteristics for the new case, the process searches the database for the most closely case who can resemble the description given. At this stage of the process it is very important provide some tools to make a refinement of the search. These tools will try to help reducing the number of cases or even display cases with just a few features of the current case (Similar cases).
b) Reuse: This process will only be active if in the retrieve phase there were similar cases that can help solve the new problem. The information from them will help solving the new problem described. The process loads the solution from the retrieved case into the new case and makes a test. If The information can solve partially the new case, the retrieved data is loaded into the new case. The next process (review) makes the necessary modifications and stores the case at the end of the retention process. However, if the case is identical, the cycle ends this process.
c) Revise: This process will only be active when the recovered case differs somewhat from current case or there are no previous similar cases. If it is similar, the differences are evaluated and the case is adapted to the new situation. If it is not similar, it is necessary to find a solution to allow the case to be stored in the repository. Another solution can be go back to the reuse process using other characteristics of the problem and see if any similar case appears.

d) Retain: This process stores the new cases that were solved on the repository so they can be used in future consultations. The system will decide which information needs to be stored and how it will be stored to facilitate future reference.

In resume, the process of CBR verifies if there is a case that is identical to that is described by the user. If not it uses the most similar case retrieved from the repository, makes small changes and tries to adapt it. If this adaptation solve the problem, the system will store the solution as a new case and in this way it will increase the system experience.

The cycle shown in Figure 5 is an exemplified process, the use of indexes with values set for its importance helps the classification and allows a better operation in the recovery and retention of cases. More information on how to implement this type of system can be obtained in the paper case-based reasoning is a methodology not a technology [25].

CONCLUSION

In this paper, it was presented an information system concept to help radiological physicians in their work. In Brazil, it is still a relative premature subject and is a new field in other countries either. However, as the discussed examples suggest, it is important to apply these techniques nowadays. Diagnoses can be made in shorter times and is possible to reduced medical errors.

The falling costs of the IT makes inevitable that the medical field will be transformed in a similar fashion as the business area. In a short time we will have an integrated system with clinic and hospital data for research and disease control. The IT sector will no longer be seen as an unnecessary cost, but as a tool that helps the business and brings benefits to physicians and patients.

The system concept generated proved to be important even for radiologists who already used to have their personnel cases records, whatever media is used for storage. The problem they face is seek information in quick and organized manner, which can be solved by the proposed information system. There are similar IS systems available in the internet [24], but they are public and the radiologists have to upload the images and enter all the information of the findings again. Also, they cannot manipulate the images because they are not in the DICOM format, something that is possible in this information system. The proposal of this system is to be an internal system in the hospital or clinic with total control by the radiology department.

In the future system recovery cases can evolve and can use more advanced techniques of CBR, becoming smarter and more useful for radiologists. The basis for the system may remain the same, since it is compatible with the DICOM standard and can easily be integrated into any IT system in the hospital. The biggest tasks to be accomplished are the standardization of the fill pattern of the exams, the semantics used when the scan is performed and the correct programming of the protocols in the system. In this way it will possible to avoid misinformation in the patient's exams. Nevertheless, this can be overcome with advanced search techniques that are widely used to search in web pages.

ACKNOWLEDGMENTS

This research was benefited by the support provided by Coppetec Foundation, through project Poli-19.257, from Federal University of Rio de Janeiro.

REFERENCES

1] A. Aamodt, E. Plaza, "Case-Based Reasoning: Foundational Issues," Methodological Variations, and System Approaches. http://citeseer. ist.psu.edu/viewdoc/download; jsessionid=29B468223A73275E9A4C0C169B5DFA5A?doi=10.1.1.15.9093&rep=rep1 &type=pdf, access on March, 10, 2011.

[2] DICOM, "Digital Imaging and Communications in Medicine." http://dicom. offis.de/index.php.en, access on June, 17, 2014.

[3] HL7 Systems and Services, "Introduction to HL7." http://www.hl7. com.au/FAQ.htm, access on March, 10, 2011.

[4] M. Rouse, "RIS - Radiology Information System." http://searchhealthit. techtarget.com/definition/Radiology-Information-System-RIS, access on March, 10, 2011.

[5] N. H. Strickland, "Picture archiving and communication system." http://www. ncbi.nlm.nih.gov/pmc/articles/PMC1718393/pdf/v083p00082.pdf, access on June, 02, 2014.

[6] J. C. de Lima, C. L. de Carvalho, "XML - Extensible Markup Language." http://www. inf.ufg.br/sites/default/files/uploads/relatorios-tecnicos/RT-INF_002-05.pdf, access on May, 28, 2014.

[7] H. Solomon, "DICOM Structured Reporting Overview." http://reportingwiki. rsna.org/images/0/00/RSNA_Reporting_Forum_Solomon.pdf, access on March, 10, 2011.

[8] Free Software Foundation Inc., GNU General Public License, version 3 (GPL-3.0). http://opensource.org/licenses/GPL-3.0, access on June, 17, 2014.

[9] Slackware Linux Inc."The Slackware Linux Project." http://www. slackware.com/, access on June, 18, 2014.

[10] Oracle Inc., "MYSQL – Open Source Database Manager." http://dev. mysql.com/doc/ refman/5.7/en/, access on June, 17, 2014.

[11] D. Evans, G. Zeilinger, U. Cappellini, "DCM4CHEE REFERENCE DOCUMENTATION Version: 2.9.1." http://www.dcm4che.org/docs/reference/ dcm4chee/pdf/dcm4chee-ref.pdf, access on March, 10, 2011.

[12] J. J. C. Portet, "Turyon Light Viewer." http://www.turyon.com/index. php, access on March, 10, 2011.

[13] R. K. Stephens, R. R. Plew, B. Morgan, J. Perkins, "SQL - Structured Query Language." http://web.ing.puc.cl/~jlortiz/Teach_Yourself_SQL_ in_21_days_FULL. pdf, access on May, 28, 2014.

[14] A. Mason, "VPNs and VPN Technologies." http://www. ciscopress. com/articles/ article.asp?p=24833, access on June, 01, 2014.

[15] D. Evans, "DCM4CHEE Database Schema Diagram." http://www.dcm4che.org/confluence/display/ee2/Database+Schema+Diagram, access on March, 10, 2011.
[16] V. Fava, "Utilizando Full-Text Search." http://www.devmedia.com.br/post-18550-Utilizando-Full-Text-Search.html, access on March, 10, 2011.
[17] K. S.Karadjl, "jpdbi - Display and optionally manipulate DCM4CHE Database entries." http://www.dcm4che.org/confluence/display/ee2/jpdbi, access on March, 10, 2011.
[18] D. Evans, "DCM2XML tool." http://www.dcm4che.org/confluence/display/d2/dcm2xml, access on March, 10, 2011.
[19] IBM Inc., Web Access to DICOM Objects (WADO) Service. http://www.research.ibm.com/haifa/projects/software/wado/, access on June, 17, 2014.
[20] D. Evans, "DCMQR tool." http://www.dcm4che.org/confluence/display/d2/dcmqr, access on March, 10, 2011.
[21] S. R. P. Soares, "Raciocínio Baseado em Casos para a Radiologia," Dissertação de Mestrado do Programa de Computação Aplicada, Universidade Estadual do Ceará, 2011. http://www.uece.br/mpcomp/index.php/arquivos/doc_download/267-dissertacao 84, access on May, 20, 2014.
[22] Bidgood WD Jr, The SNOMED DICOM microglossary: controlled terminology resource for data interchange in biomedical imaging. http://www.ncbi.nlm.nih.gov/pubmed/9865038, access on November, 28, 2014.
[23] DICOM, CP 722 Add Cross-reference between Body Part Examined and Anatomic Region. ftp://medical.nema.org/medical/dicom/final/cp722_ ft.pdf, access on October, 11, 2014.
[24] MedPix - Search and Browse Proven Cases. http://rad.usuhs.edu/medpix/parent.php3?mode=search, access on July, 07, 2015.
[25] WATSON, Ian. Case-based reasoning is a methodology not a technology, AI-CBR, University of Salford (1999). http://citeseerx.ist.psu.edu/viewdoc/download?doi=10.1.1.129.9508&rep=rep1&type=pdf, access on July, 19, 2015.

In: Models and Methods for Supporting Decision-Making … ISBN: 978-1-63485-173-2
Editors: Carlos N. Bouza, Flávio L. de Mello et al.

Chapter 10

Design of Routes for Waste Collection: Centro Habana's Case Study

Joanna Campbell Amos * ***and Sira Allende Alonso***
Mathematics and Computation Faculty,
University of Havana, Cuba

Abstract

Waste management deals with the collection, transport and disposal of the solid waste. In recent years waste management has become a problem worldwide due to population growth (especially in urban areas), the environmental effects of residues accumulation and the progressive increment of the costs in waste management. Hence, municipalities need to improve solid waste management. In particular, it is important to reduce the distance travelled by the collection vehicles. Routes design for collecting domiciliary residues can be modeled as arc-edge routing problem on a mixed graph, the Mixed Chinese Postman's Problem (MCPP). MCPP is a NP-Hard problem in contrast with the –Chinese Postman´s Problem on directed and undirected graphs (CPP). This work deals with the routes design of domiciliary residues using the implementation of a new heuristic for MCCP. The use of the system for designing the collection routes in a municipality of Havana, Cuba is described.

Keywords: CPP, MCPP, SA, Route Design, Solid Waste

Introduction

Large cities have big volumes of garbage. Its collection and disposal at adequate points is an important issue due to the impact that the residuals has for the health and the environment. Indeed, pollution by toxic substances disposed in wrong places have caused the contamination of rivers, soils, with the corresponding consequences for the human welfare.

---

* Corresponding Author address: Email:joanna@matcom.uh.cu, Email:sira@matcom.uh.cu.

That is why many countries have increased the budget dedicated to the gathering of the garbage. Research devoted to optimize this process have appeared, specifically to the management of the solid residuals and to examine the relationship cost-effectiveness and the impact in the environment, in terms of routing design for solid waste collection. For Computational techniques are important tools for improving the design of the routes, see [3]. To achieve a good design of the garbage collection routes it is necessary to consider all the following aspects:

1) The design of routes should increase the productivity, that is the distance where garbage is collected.
2) The routes should not be divided neither overlapped. Each one should their own trucks.
3) The beginning of a route should be near the starting point and the end near the place of final disposition of residuals.
4) In places with level differences it is desirable that the route should starts at the highest places and ends at the lowest part.
5) The traffic regulations shall be taken into account.
6) To avoid the turns to the left and the U-turns in order to reduce the driver´s effort on performing his job.

It is also necessary to know the characteristics of the zone in order that the routes of the trucks of garbage may not cause problems, as traffic jams, see [4].

In Cuba the solid waste collection is a problem which is not yet well solved, particularly in the capital, Havana. Its complexity is increased by the economical limitations, typical of Third World countries, and the condition of country blocked economically and technologically.

Havana, with more than two million inhabitants, generates around 17,000m^3 of solid wastes on a daily basis; for municipality, the average ranges between 1,000 and 2,000m^3 [1, 2, 12, 15]. The garbage collection is made by the Group Servicios Comunales. Diverse transportation means are used including animal traction. Assuming that the motorized vehicles have a capacity of eleven tons and average consumption of seven liters of fuel by travel, one hundred trips would be needed to transfer urban solid waste to the dumping sites and 700 l. of fuel would be consumed. Around 560000g of CO_2 would be generated, a considerable volume of pollution [2, 12].

To eliminate garbage accumulation on the streets the city needs more bins and vehicles for the collection. The current stage is characterized by material lacks and organizational difficulties The collection fleet has 62 trucks, 48 of them, belonging to the Provincial Unit of Hygiene, 15 have breaks damage, 33 have transitory affectation. It is necessary to supply the lack of infrastructure, technologies, planning and control of the activities in the management of the solid residuals. Nowadays, the collection routes are designed in an intuitive way. On other side, there are waste accumulation in different points, forcing the trucks to stop more times and to travel longer distances than those contemplated in the original route, with the consequent increment of time and fuel consumption [1, 15].

The budget of Servicios Comunales is up to 170.6 million pesos, plus the expenses related with the fuel, and the acquisition of specialized instruments for the deposit and the collection of the garbage. Only budget dedicated to Health and Education are higher than the budget dedicated to management [1].

In this work we present the use of a new heuristic for solving MCCP. It is implemented in our system VisualCPPSolver and applicable to the design of routes for collecting domiciliary residues. VisualCPPSolver, solves the MCPP, the algorithm is based on the metaheuristic Simulating Annealing (SA). The geographic data for the graph has been obtained from a Geographic Information System. *Centro Habana* is the municipality of Havana chosen as case study. Some streets of *Centro Habana* are one-way and other ones are two-way, the problem is modeled as a MCPP. *Centro Habana* is one of the municipality of highest garbage generators a most densely populated of Cuba.

This chapter is organized as follows, in section 1 we present the MCCP mathematical model that is used to perform the problem over the selected areas of garbage collection. In section 2 we consider the Simulated Annealing algorithm used to deal with the problem. In section 3, the numerical results corresponding to the application of VisualCPPSolver to the selected instances are shown.

MODELING POSTMAN ROUTE FOR MIXED GRAPHS

In the literature, the design of the routes for the solid waste collection is mostly modeled as Capacitated Arc Routing problems (CARP) or as a Capacitated Vertex Routing problems (CVRP). The type of model depends on the type of service. If the collection service is residential, it is a problem of routes on arcs. On the other hand, if there are some points where the garbage is concentrated such as commercial or industrial centers or by bins, it will be modeled as a vertex routing problem. The capacities are given by the amount of garbage which is collected at the arcs or nodes. Of course if the capacity of the trucks is large enough and can collect all the garbage of the sector, the model reduces to a Traveling Salesman Problem.

Central property in the study of CPP, is the Eulerian property. A connected graph is said to be Eulerian if there exists a closed walk in G containing each arc exactly once and each vertex at least once. A fundamental result is the statement of necessary and sufficient conditions for a connected graph to be Eulerian [5]:

- If G is undirected, every vertex must have an even degree, i.e., and an even number of incident edges;
- If G is directed, the number of arcs entering and leaving each vertex must be equal;
- If G is mixed, every vertex must be incident to an even number of directed and undirected arcs; moreover, for every $S \subseteq V$, the difference between the number of directed arc from S to V\S and the number of directed arcs from V\S to S must be less than or equal to the number of undirected arc joining S and V\S. This condition is called “balanced set condition,” [6].

The mathematical model for a MCPP proposed by Kapauff and Koehler [7] is the following [7]:

$$\text{(MCPP)Minimize} \sum_{<v_i,v_j>\in A} c_{ij}x_{ij} + \sum_{<v_i,v_j>\in E^+} c_{ij}x_{ij} + \sum_{<v_i,v_j>\in E^-} c_{ij}x_{ij} \quad (1)$$

Subject to:

$$\sum_{i=1}^{n} x_{ij} - \sum_{i=1}^{n} x_{ji} = 0 \ \forall j \in V \quad (2)$$

$$x_a \geq 1 \ \forall a \in A \quad (3)$$

$$x_{e^+} + x_{e^-} \geq 1 \ \forall e \in E \quad (4)$$

$$x_l \in Z \ \forall l \in A \cup E^+ \cup E^- \quad (5)$$

The objective function minimizes the cost to add arcs or edges in one sense (E^+) and /or other (E^-) The restriction (2) guarantees the Eulerian property. The restrictions (3) guarantee that the arcs are visited at least once. Constraints (4) express that the edges should be passed at least once in one or the two possible senses. The restrictions (5) express the number of times that the arcs/edges were added to the solution.

This problem was considered by a many authors. Nobert et al. [8] considered another integer programming model and a solution algorithm for solving the problem. The proposed approach uses the Simplex method to obtain sharp lower bounds by solving successive relaxations of the model. Optimality is achieved by using Gomory cuts, blossom inequalities and balanced set constraints. Most recently, Negreiros et al. [9] proposed a hybrid Branch and Bound method considering the metaheuristic GRASP for obtaining an upper bound of the objective function and reducing computation time. It was implemented in the software XNES and tested in different instances. Corberán et al. [10] proposed a GRASP heuristic to the MCPP, with good results for a number of selected instances. The use of the metaheuristic Simulated Annealing (SA) has not been reported in the consulted literature. In the next section we describe the basic ideas of a heuristic algorithm inspired in this metaheuristic for solving MCPP.

Simulated Annealing for the MCPP

The following diagram shows the structure of SA used in the heuristic to solve MCPP.

An initial feasible solution is built following the idea proposed by Coberán [10]. The edges are oriented considering semi degrees of the vertices of the graph in order to obtain a directed graph on which an algorithm for solving the Chinese Postman's Problem on directed graph is applied. After the initial solution obtained, a new solution is built maintaining the Eulerian property.

A necessary condition for the existence of Eulerian tour is the symmetry of the graph. In the proposed algorithm, start solution and all the solutions generated are symmetric multigraphs. Movements from a solution to another neighbor solution are described by the orientation assigned to the edges and the addition of arcs/edges oriented to the graph. As result, an Eulerian directed multi-graph is obtained. The objective function to evaluate on each multigraph, is the cost of the Eulerian tour.

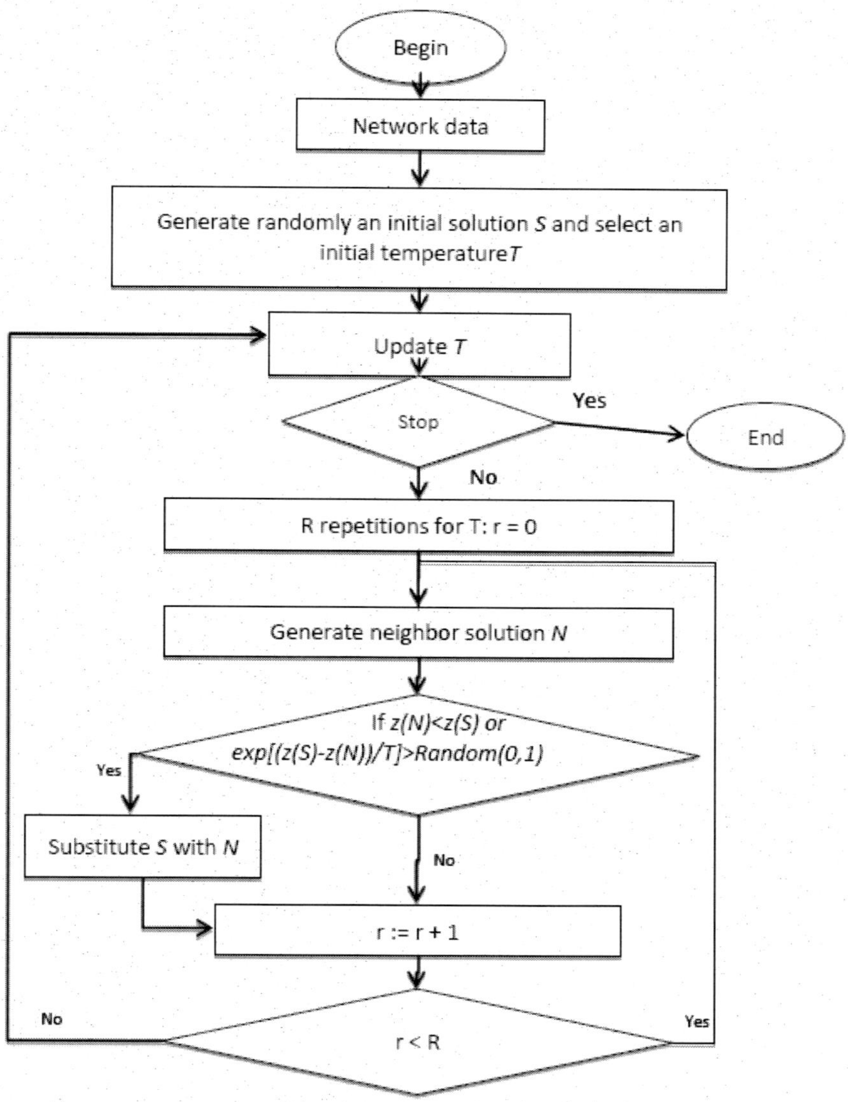

Figure 1. SA general schema for the MCPP.

A neighborhood of a solution is built changing the orientation of one of its edges. After this change on edge $< v_1, v_2 >$, the out-degree and in-degree of two vertices are not equal ($|d^+(v_i) - d^-(v_i)|=2$). Therefore, feasibility condition is not satisfied, and, the graph is no longer Eulerian. We must find two paths in graph from v_1 to v_2 and add them into an augmented graph to recuperate the degree conditions of both vertex. Figure 2 shows the neighborhood criterion.

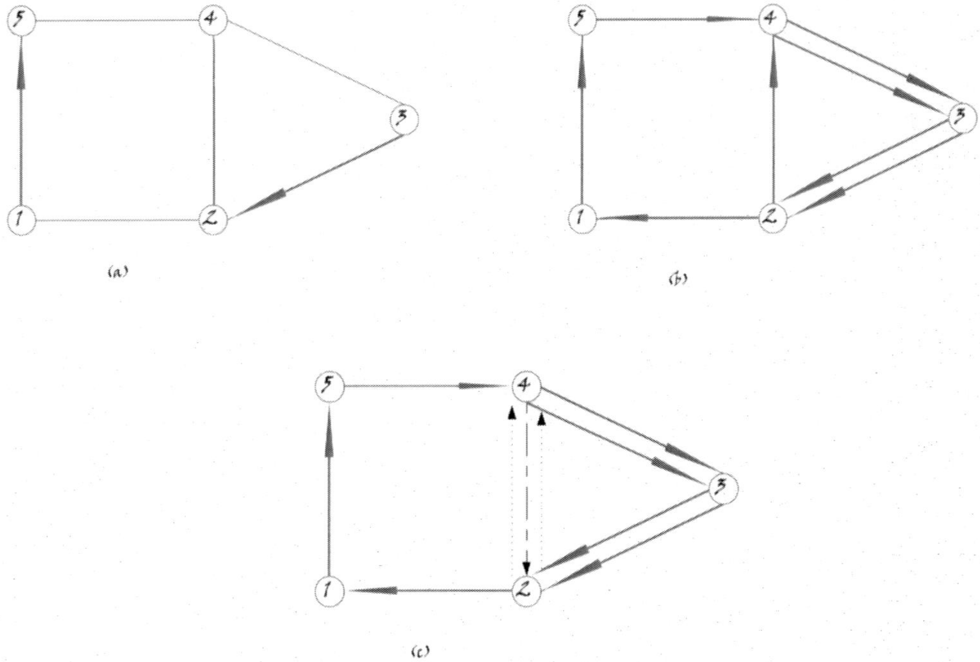

Figure 2. (a) The original graph; (b) The graph increased where the edge (2.4) is oriented 2 -> 4; (c) The direction of the edge (2,4) is reversed and the paths 2 → 4 and 2 → 4 are added to the original graph.

It is possible that the neighborhood criterion introduce redundancies since they may add new paths. If we find a cycle in the augmented graph and remove it, we must check if the solution is still valid. Figure 3 shows the redundancy elimination.

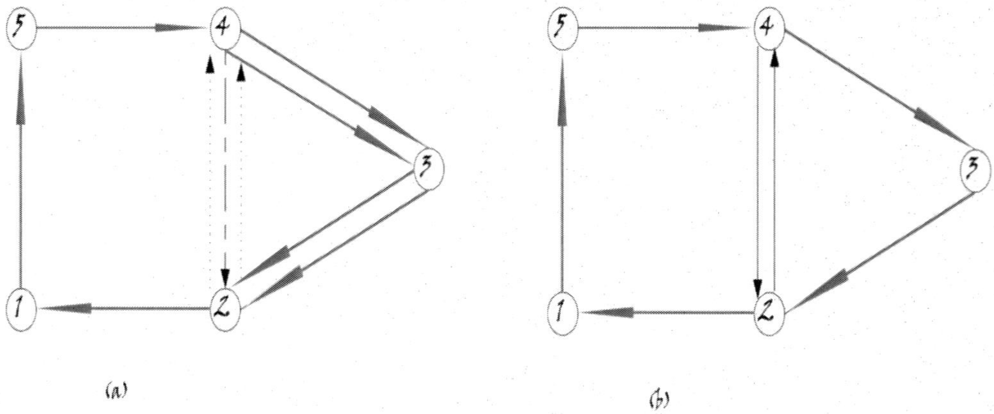

Figure 3. (a) The neighbor solution obtained by changing the direction of an edge with the cycle 2 → 4 → 3 → 2; (b) the result of the elimination graph cycle.

The heuristic is implemented in the tool VISUALCPPSOLVER. It allows the application for designing collection routes as it is showed in the following sections.

THE VISUALCPPSOLVER

Visualcppsolver is a software for solving the CPP on undirected, directed and mixed graphs. It has been implemented on the .NET platform, version 3.5, and programming language C#. It has a modular structure.

First the graph is loaded. It is stored in a .grf file with the syntaxis of graph produced by the XNES software [9]. The application allows its visualization.

Once the graph is shown, we can obtain information associated to the graph like the graph type (directed, not directed, mixed), number of vertices, arcs, edges, perimeter of the graph (the sum of the costs of the edges/arcs). For the mixed case it is allowed to configure the parameters for the Simulating Annealing.

After ending the execution of the algorithm for MCPP, the results are reported and they can be visualized in the area.

In Figure 4, the tools of VisualCPPSolver are shown:

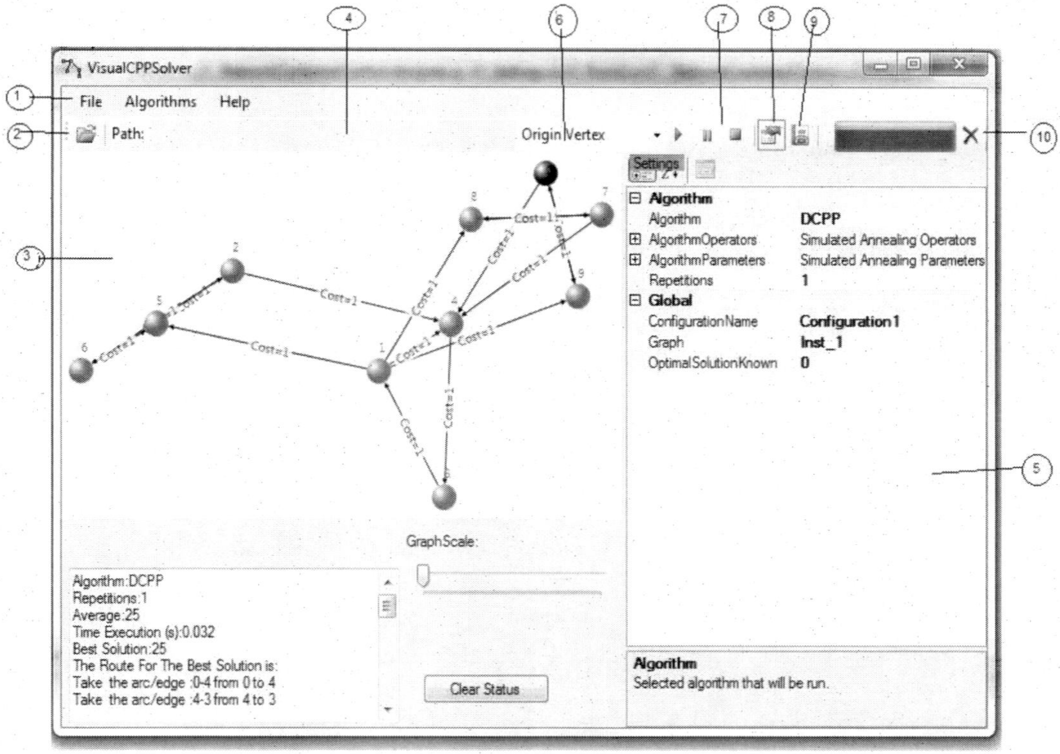

Figure 4. Overview of the main application window VisualCPPSolver

The meaning of the numbers are the following:

1. The Main menu of the application has three parts:
    - File menu lets the user open a new network, close and save the current network and exit the application.

- Algorithms menu allows to describe the selected instance, to create a new one and the random generation of new instances.
- Help menu displays a window with instruction about the application.

2. Open button on the toolbar: closes the current file and opens a new option. It is a shortcut to the Open option of the File menu.
3. Display area of the input data: place where the graph stored in the .grf file or randomly generated file is displayed. The black node represents the initial vertexwhere the closed route on the graph will begin (by default the first vertex will be considered the initial node). The other nodes are drawn in red. The arches/edges represent the connections between nodes of the graph and are drawn in black.
4. Address Bar: Displays physical disk location of the open file.
5. Configuration control: allows the modification of the parameters of the heuristic algorithm for MCPP.
6. Control for changing the initial node where the tour begins.
7. Execution buttons.
   - Run button: starts the execution of the algorithm with the parameters set given in the Configuration control.
   - Pause button: pause execution.
   - Stop button: completely stops the execution of the algorithm.
8. Settings button: shows or hides the control parameter settings used mainly for the mixed case.
9. Report button: shows or hides the window reports.
10. Close button: close the current network.

CASE STUDY: CENTRO HABANA

In this section, we discuss a case study in order to show the application in the routing design for the waste collection.

The municipality of Centro Habana with high population density generates a lot of garbage. The map of Centro Habana, distances and traffic orientation of the blocks were obtained from OpenStreetMap [11]. We consider the zone divided into two collection sectors, (see Figure 5). In both sectors there are one-way and two way streets, hence the sectors can be modeled as mixed graphs. A set of trucks have been assigned to each sector every service day.

The graph associated to each sector or instances was obtained using the application XNES [9]. Information on traffic direction and distance associated to each arc or edges is obtained from OpenStreetMap [11]. Arc´s direction is fixed according of the traffic direction.

The instances were run in VisualCPPSolver to obtain routes with small length. Tests were performed on a computer with Intel Core 2 Duo T8100 @ 2.10 GHz procesor, 4.00 GB of RAM, operating system Windows 7 64-bit.

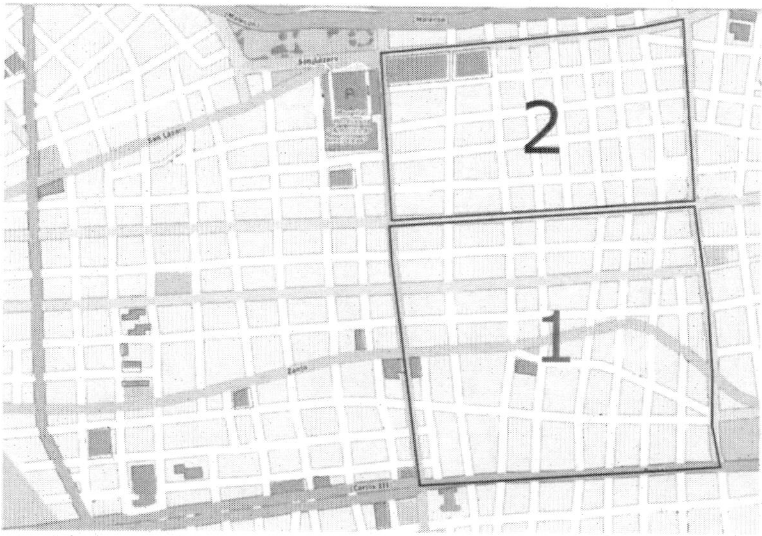

Figure 5. Visualization of Centro Habana and its two sectors.

The characteristics of each sector and the routes designed by VisualCPPSolver are the following:

Sector 1 covers 56 blocks with a perimeter of 8,423 m. Figure 6 shows the mixed graph associated to sector 1 obtained by XNES. The graph has 74 vertex, 70 arcs and 59 edges.

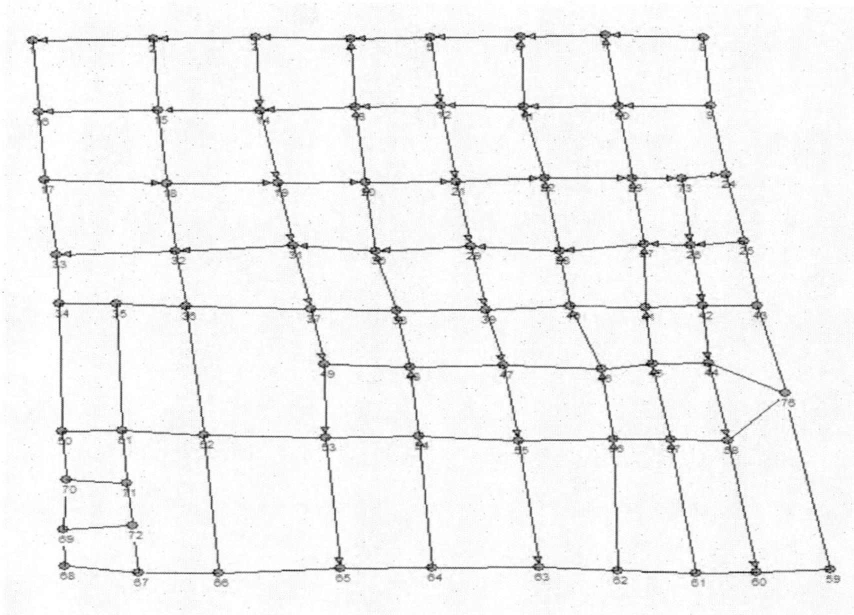

Figure 6. Mixed Graph associated to sector 1 of Centro Habana.

The route designed by VisualCPPSolver for the sector 1 has a length of 9,946m. It has been obtained 84s. Figure 7 shows the multi-graph route description over the map of Centro Habana-sector 1.

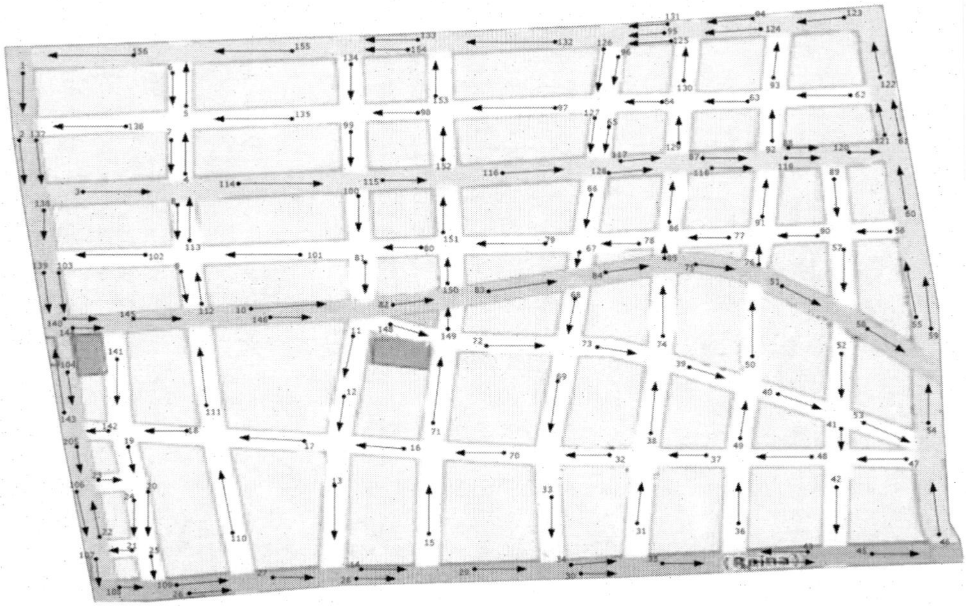

Figure 7. Route description on the map for the sector 1.

Sector 2 coverss 41 blocks. It has a perimeter of 6,691m. Figure 8 shows the mixed graph associated to sector 2 obtained by XNES. The graph has 55 vertex, 33 arcs and 62 edges.

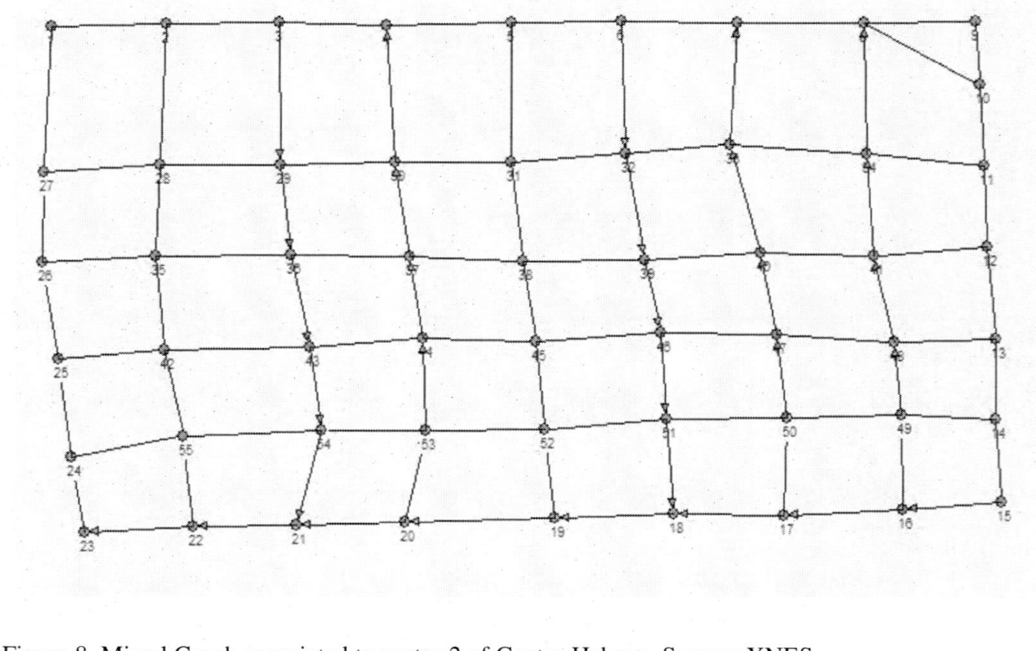

Figure 8. Mixed Graph associated to sector 2 of Centro Habana. Source: XNES.

The route designed this case has a length of 7,988m. This solution was obtained in 30s, by VisualCPPSolver. Figure 9 shows the route over the map.

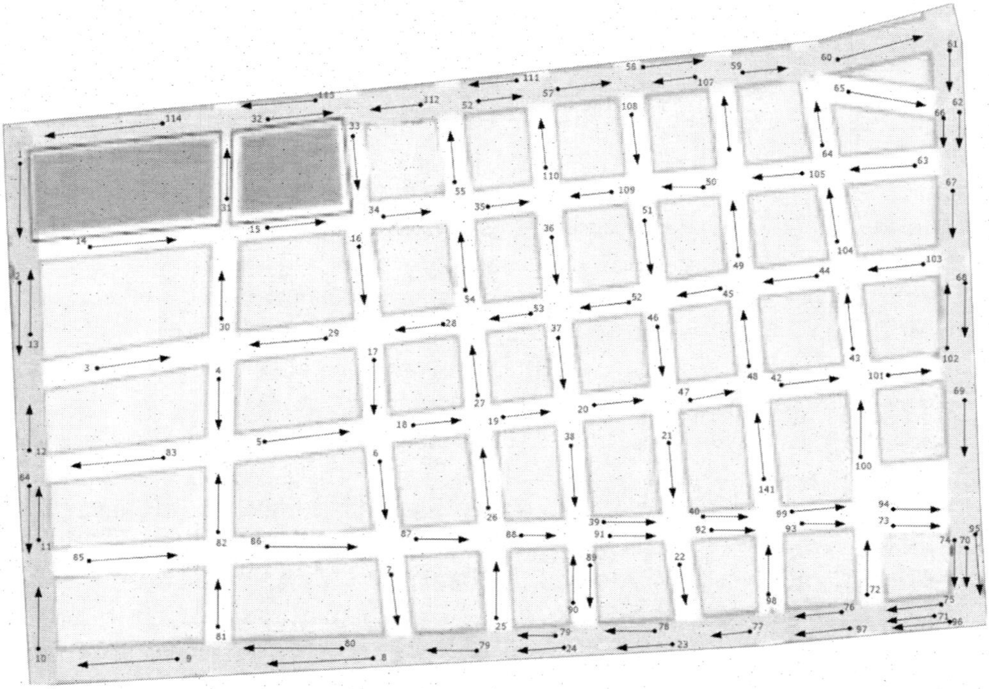

Figure 9. Route description on the map for the sector 2.

Conclusion and Recommendations

Management of urban residues has a big impact in human health and environment. It requires however, considerable inversions. It is necessary to analyze the relationship cost-effectiveness of the services. Vehicles for waste collection are expensive and fuel consumers. Hence, a rational design of the collection routes is very important, particularly in Cuba.

In this chapter, we have presented the application of a computational tool (VisualCPPSolver) to design waste collection routes. Kern of the tool is the solution of Chinese Postman´s (CPP) Problem on undirected, directed and mixed graph. To solve the problem on mixed graph, a heuristic is proposed.

To illustrate the use of VisualCPPSolver, a central municipality of Havana with two collection sectors has been chosen. It was modeled as Chinese Postman´s Problem on mixed graph (MCPP). The proposed heuristic for MCPP has needed an execution time inferior to 2 minutes for given the routes.

As future research lines, it is planned the inclusion of other constraints (on travel time, time windows etc.) and the exchange with municipalities authorities about their requirement and results of the computational tool. It would be also interesting to consider the use of the software to design the routes of fumigation against vectors of dangerous diseases.

REFERENCES

[1] Análisis Sectorial de Residuos Sólidos en Cuba. *No. 13 OPS/OMS.*

[2] Palacios, F., Garcia, E., Garcia, O., Fraguela, V., Ruiz, A., Sarduy, M.C., Potrillé, F., (2001) Manejo de residuos sólidos urbanos en la zona litoral de laBahía de la habana. *Informe. Cimab. La Habana. 50 p.*

[3] Nuortioa, T., Kytöjokib, J., Niskaa, H. and Bräysy, O. (2005). Improved Route Planning and Scheduling of Waste Collection and Transport. *Operations Research.*

[4] SEDESOL. (1999). *Manual de Técnicas Administrativas para el Servicio de limpia Municipal.* Mexico: Ingenieria para el Control de Residuos Municipales e Industriales S.A de C.V.D.F Mexico.

[5] Eiselt, H. and Laporte, G. (1995). Arc routing problems, part II the rural postman problem. *Operations Research.*

[6] Nobert, Y. and Picard, J.-c. (1996). An optimal algorithm for the mixed Chinese postman problem. *Networks, 27(2), 97.*

[7] Kappauf, C.H.; Koehler (1979) - The mixed postman problem. *Discrete Applied Mathematics 1, 89-103.*

[8] Nobert, Y.; Picard, J-C (1996) - An optimal algorithm for the Mixed Chinese Portman *Problem. Networks 27, 95-108.*

[9] Negreiros, M., Junior, W., Palhano, A., Coutinho, E., Castro, G., Negreiros, F.J., Barcelos, G., Rezende, B., Pereira, L., O Problema do Carteiro Chinês, Algoritmos Exatos e um Ambiente MVI para Análise de suas Instâncias: Sistema XNês, *Pesquisa Operacional, v.29, n.2, p.323-363, Maio a Agosto de 2009.*

[10] Corberán, A.; Martí, J.M. and Sanchis, J.M. (2002). A GRASP heuristic for the mixed Chinese Postman problem. *European Journal of Operational Research, 142, 70-80.*

[11] Devsaran: OpenStreetMap SDK for .NET/Mono. www.osmSharp.com.

[12] Cardoso, M. G., C., O. and N. H, M. J. (2009). Experiencia piloto para el manejo integral de los residuos sólidos urbanos en localidades con características urbanas y semi urbanas. Caso de estudio en ciudad de La Habana, Cuba. *Mapping Interativo.*

[13] Goldberg, A. V. and Tarjan, R. E. (1989.). Finding Minimum-Cost Circulations by Canceling Negative Cycles. *Journal of the ACM, 36(4):873–886.*

[14] Evans, J. and Minieka, E. (1992). Optimization Algorithms for Networks and Graphs. *Marcel Dekker Inc, New York, 278-315.*

[15] Alberty Loforte Arlin, Tras el Rastro de la basura. Arlin internet@gramma.cu 11 de Diciembre del 2014.

In: Models and Methods for Supporting Decision-Making … ISBN: 978-1-63485-173-2
Editors: Carlos N. Bouza, Flávio L. de Mello et al.

Chapter 11

COMPARISON METHODS OF DIGITAL ELEVATION MODEL CORRECTION, IN THE SUBWATERSHED V ANIVERSARIO, CUYAGUATEJE BASIN CUBA

Yeleine Almoza Hernández[1,*], Abdiel Fernández Alvarez[1], Yasser Vázquez[1] and Andrea Petroseli[2]

[1]Departamento Física-Matemática, Facultad Ciencias Técnicas, Universidad Agraria de la Habana, Cuba
[2]DAFNE Department, Tuscia University, Italy

ABSTRACT

For several decades, the terrain topography has been studied in depth due to its importance and influence in other disciplines, like vegetation sciences, territorial planning, hydrology and others. Digital Elevation Model (DEM) data as the others raster data, is a matrix of cells regularly spaced, where the attribute is the elevation datum, usually measured at particular ground positions and later interpolated in order to reconstruct the whole matrix of cells. Digital Elevation Models are useful because, from them, we can obtain other interesting data. Consequently, we consider helpful the continuous efforts to gain a better understanding of the preprocessing techniques aiming to correct Digital Elevation Models. For these reasons, the aim of the present research work is to analyze the geomorphological transformations produced by three DEMs correction methods in the particular scenario of V Aniversario subwatershed, Cuyaguateje River. For this analysis, the following correction methods have been selected: Fill method because is the most widely used in literature; TOPAZ method, which combines fills and cut; and finally, the physically based method PEM4PIT. The results shows the capabilities of mathematical methods (TOPAZ and Fill) over physicallys based method PEM4PIT, to correct depression getting the best final correlation with the original DEM, in doing so creating less errors introduction for further works based on DEMs. TOPAZ seems preferable to correct basins with high particular geomorphic characteristics like the research study area.

* Email: yeleinealmoza82@gmail.com.

Keywords: elevation datum, transformations, geomorphological

INTRODUCTION

The development of aerospace and computer technologies in recent decades has taken a turn for Geosciences. Obtaining aerial and satellite images with higher resolution and more powerful computers and software for processing, today allow a deeper and more detailed understanding of our planet. An example is the Digital Elevation Models (DEM). These are available with resolutions from low to medium, to very high, from aerial photographs, satellite imagery, optical and radar or LIDAR technology (Light Detection and Ranging; acronym in English) according [1]. However, despite technological advances, it is well known that it is not possible to obtain a free DEM of holes, depressions or flat areas. These features can be faithful representations of the land or errors caused by different causes: (1) methods of acquisition and production of DEMs such as remote sensing, due to properties of the sensors, biased reflectance values or to convert vector data from raster format elevations; (2) truncated data to interpolate decimal values to integers according to authors [2, 3, 4]. In the field of hydrology, has shown that even in the DEM obtained with LIDAR technology, where the resolution becomes an order of magnitude less than the most frequently used in hydrological modeling, application of the latest models may return incorrect results, if not adequately treated eliminating depressions and flat areas [5].

There are several methods of correction DEMs. The most frequently used, is called Filling and Flooding (hereinafter Filling) [2], which considers all depressions as model errors relief and consists of filling the depressions to the height of the child from neighbors. This method has been implemented in Geographical Information System (GIS) software, such as commercial (ArcGIS) and non-commercial (GRASS) software, containing packages for digital terrain analysis. In other cases, the depressions are understood as a result of the estimation and/or overestimation of the elevation, thus assuming the possibility of closed depressions are the result of the creation of false walls and not only false gaps. On this occasion, the solution lies in the combination of 'breach' and/or 'fill in residual depression,' and has been implemented in the "Topographic Parameterization" software (hereinafter Topaz) according authors [6]. The methods mentioned are strictly geometric, but in the literature can be found others, such as modeling physical basis, which simulate natural processes such as erosion. An example is the method of physical basis "Physically based Erosion Model for PIT filling" (hereinafter PEM4PIT) [3]. There are other methods that have been developed for the correction of digital elevation models like [7, 8]. In literature you can find comparisons between any of these methods with respect to the standard method Filling [9, 10, 4, 8, 5]. Moreover, it has not been defined the method given for each geometry hydrological basin or determination process, so it is considered useful to devote efforts to better understand the preprocessing techniques aimed at correcting DEM. Because each method assumes its own considerations on the origin of depressions, mathematical methods and algorithms, one can understand that the selection of either involves individual characterizations of watercourses, earrings and other parameters that define the hydraulic behavior and a hydrological basin. In the present work has as objective to make a comparison of geomorphological changes produced by three methods MDE correction of subwatershed V Anniversary, Cuyaguateje River.

Several natural sciences, from geomorphology to vegetation sciences, have been showing an increasing interest in applications based on the accurate representation of topography as provided by the most recent digital elevation models (DEMs) [11, 12, 13, 14]. The detailed reconstruction of the environment is required to simulate at best different physical processes, hence many techniques have been developed in the last years to obtain DEMs with resolution from low to very high, as airborne data digital photogrammetry, airborne Light Detection and Ranging (LiDAR) – Derived Elevation Data, satellite radar altimetry, etc., [1]. It is worth noting, therefore, that regardless of data source, a DEM is the result of both measurements and mathematical and/or statistical processes to the information, where each record possibility that all representations are correct according [15]: indeed, in every DEM, a series of errors are present, due to several reasons; from the elevation data truncation when interpolating floating point values to integer precision, to the interpolation algorithms when converting vector-based elevation information, such as contour lines, into a gridded format. These procedures lead to the situation that is common to find in DEMs a single cell or a continuous area that has a lower elevation than its entire neighbouring areas, generating what is called a sink, pit or depression area. When geomorphic applications dealing with the reconstruction of the surface water flow movement are addressed, such as hydrological or hydraulic applications, these features cause an interruption of downstream flow movement through the DEM, affecting every posterior modelling or analysis [3, 1, 5]: this circumstance is obviously due to the inability of the existing flow routing schemes to determine a way for the water to move downward from an area having elevation lower than the surrounding one. It has been confirmed that even the applications of the more recent hydrological models can provide incorrect results when performed with the most detailed DEMs, if depressions and flat areas are not adequately addressed [5].

Many algorithms have been implemented to deal with this issue, based on different considerations with regard to depressions nature and the adopted mathematical procedures. The simplest case considers all depressions as errors produced by underestimation of elevation. The most widely used algorithm is based on this idea, and the correction method consists of raising the depression until reaching the elevation of the lower surrounding neighbour. Known with the acronym Fill or Filling according to [2], this method has been implemented in the most widely used commercial geographic information system (GIS) packages, as GIS softwares ESRI ArcInfo, ArcGIS, and the open source Unixbased GRASS. In other cases, the depressions are seen as the result of underestimation and/or overestimation, assuming the possibility that closed depressions are consequences of creating false walls. This time, the correction method consists in combining ‘cut the wall’ and/or ‘fill remaining depression areas,’ and is implemented in the software “Topographic Parameterization” (TOPAZ) [6]. Both the aforementioned methods are strictly geometric, but in literature there are also the physically based methods, where natural processes, for instance erosion, are simulated by mathematical procedures to perform the DEM correction. One example is the physically based method Physically based Erosion Model for PIT filling (PEM4PIT) [3]. Some other cases consist in applying a combination of various above mentioned methods [7] or perform local surface interpolation by the authors [16]. A different kind of method considers all depressions as natural and a good representation of landscape, and the correction method is the redirection of downstream flow until reaching the basin outlet, without producing any change in the topography, but forcing the river network delineation [8].

Many methods have been developed; however, usually they are applied in literature without considering the influences over the geomorphological conditions. Indeed, different methods assume different considerations about depression's nature, mathematical procedures and algorithms, so the modeller can understand that the selection of a specific correction method involves particular characterization of flow paths, and consequent modifications in hydrological or hydraulic analysis according [17]. About that, some results illustrate advantages of certain correction methods for particular analysis and/or particular basin topographic conditions, in particular in terms of the consequent hydrogeomorphological modelling [3, 4, 10, 17]. At present, however, the literature has not well defined suitable methods for each context. Therefore, we consider useful the continuous efforts to gain a better understanding of the preprocessing techniques aiming to correct DEMs. For these reasons, the aim of the present work is to analyze the geomorphological transformations produced by three DEM correction methods in one scenario. For this analysis, the following correction methods have been selected: Fill, the most widely used in literature; TOPAZ, which combines fills and cut; and finally, the physically based method PEM4PIT. The employed methods have been chosen because in literature it is common to find comparisons between the standard Filling procedure, i.e., the most used DEM correction method implemented in several software packages, and a second procedure, often more advanced but also less diffuse, while it is uncommon to have comparisons among many different techniques at the same moment and in the same geomorphologic conditions.

Study Area, as above mentioned, a Cuban subwatershed was selected, characterized by very different hydrological and geomorphic conditions with other subwatershed in the Pinar del Rio Province. The Cuban basin, V Aniversario (Figure1), is a location of agricultural and economical interest with an area of 131.21km^2. The region contains one of the most peculiar geographic formations of Cuba, named "Mogotes," a term used for karst hills typically rounded by tower-like forms and surrounded by nearly flat alluvial plains. This basin is under a typically tropical climate with an average temperature of 25.1ºC and a yearly cumulative precipitation of 1770 mm.

The V Aniversario DEM has been obtained firstly with the cartographic sheet digitalization (Contour Line) see Figure 2. Then it was interpolated with kriging in ArcGIS 9.2, data from a 1:10000-elevation map, resulting in a 25 × 25 m resolution digital elevation model. Our interest resides with the morphological characteristics of this basin.

V Aniversario combines large flat areas, hills and the Mogotes. These conditions constitute a challenge for preprocessing techniques, testing the possibilities of the methods to deal, for example, with slope changes, especially around the Mogotes' edges, which tend to be nearly vertical. On the other hand, there are large natural closed depressions in that basin, whose treatment could represent a source of error introduction.

As it was mentioned previously three methods were selected, now we will explain with more detail in that consist: Fill [2]; TOPAZ [6]; and PEM4PIT [3], whose characteristics are briefly described below. The selection was made considering differences in considering the nature of depressions and the treatment of pit and flat areas. The Fill method is the most widely used for hydrological applications. It has been implemented in the majority of GIS software packages, such as proprietary GIS softwares ESRI ArcInfo, ArcGIS 9.2, as well as the open source Unixbased GRASS. Here, pits and depressions are considered all fake, and a result of underestimation of the elevation at certain points. All depressions, therefore, are filled to the elevation of the minor neighbour, as shown in Figure 3.

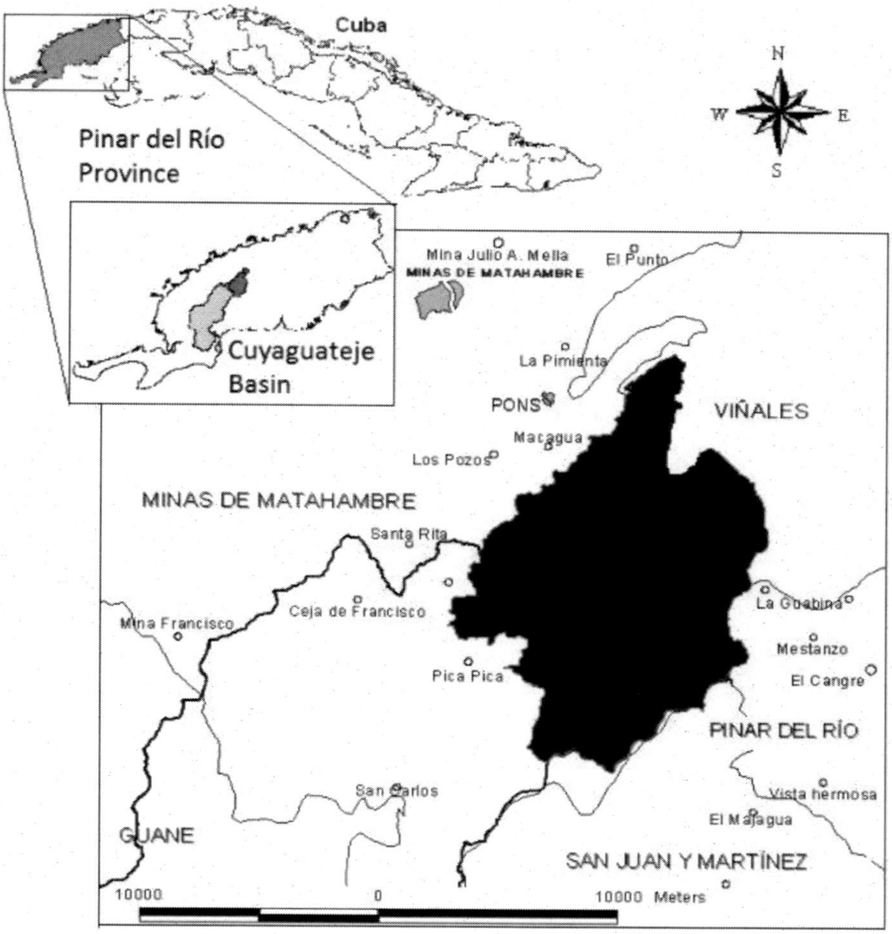

Figure 1. V Aniversario subwatershed location.

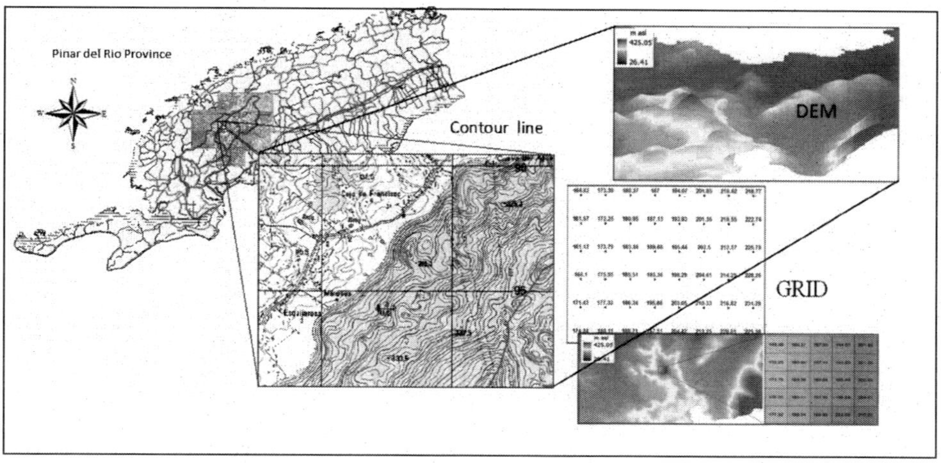

Figure 2. Contour line used to make DEM from digitalization in ArcGIS 9.2.

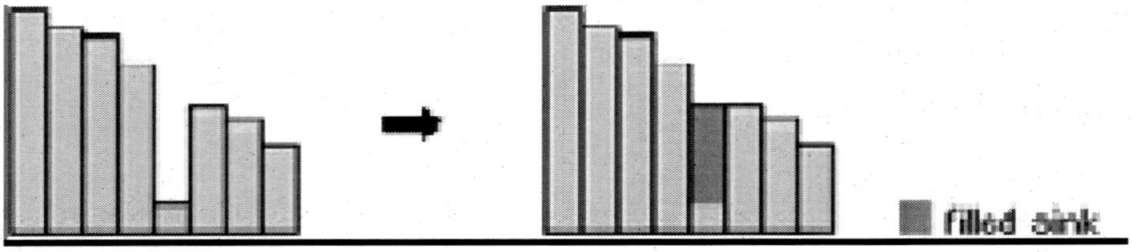

Figure 3. Lateral profile of depression before and after the *Fill* application (from ArcInfohelp guide).

The second selected method was TOPAZ [6]. In this case, all depressions are considered as spurious points, resulting from underestimation and/or overestimation of the elevation. This consideration involves both possibilities, the occurrence of sinks by underestimation of elevation at certain points, as well as the presence of closed depressions, generated by a false wall for overestimation of height at some cell(s). The proposed solution consists in three steps. Firstly, the points where is not possible the flow direction assignment, and having at least one neighbour cell with high elevation, are flagged. This step permits the separation of inflow sinks and flat areas, avoiding the treatment and consequently the breaching of plane areas. The corresponding contributing area at each inflow sink is determined. If some cell edge of the inflow-sink contributing area has lower elevation neighbours on both, inside and outside, this area will be consider as a closed depression to be breached. The breaching algorithm is the second step. The cell edges adjacent to a lower elevation cell outside the contributing area are selected as potential outlets. If more than one potential outlet was identified, then the one with the lowest elevation is selected. If the lowest elevation is shared, it will be selected as the one with the steepest slope out of the contributing area. Following these criteria, breaching is permitted only through an area of higher elevation that separates two areas of lower elevation. In addition, the breaching length is limited to a maximum value of two cells, in order to avoid breaching of any possible actual topographic feature. In case of fulfilling all conditions, the breaching takes place, else the depression is simply filled. After the breaching process, some closed depressions, might only be reduced, remaining partially unchanged. To complete the correction process, the remaining depressions, as well as depressions where the breaching was not possible, are filled. The TOPAZ filling procedure raises the elevation of cells inside the depression to the selected outlet elevation value. After that, the flat areas are treated adding infinitesimally small values to the elevation at some cells, enough to be understood by computer algorithms during the assignment of flow direction [9]. Adding values of 10^{-5} order, the elevations are incremented to generate into the filled area gradients toward lower terrain. The result is a DEM without zero slope areas, where the flow direction can be defined at every cell. For further details, consult [9] and [6].

The physically based erosion model for pit and flat areas removal, PEM4PIT, proposes a different solution. The following simplified physically based landscape evolution equation is implemented:

$$0 = U - \beta A^{\theta} S + D\nabla^2 z \qquad (1)$$

where U is the tectonic uplift rate, $\beta A^{\theta} S$ is the fluvial incision term, $D\nabla^2 z$ represents the erosion or deposition rate by diffusive processes depending on landscape shape, A is the contributing area at the site, θ is the scaling slope–area coefficient, β is the surface erodibility, and D is the hillslope diffusivity [3]. This method simulates the topographic surface evolution assuming equilibrium between the tectonic uplift and the sediment flows produced by fluvial erosion and overland diffusion. The model is able to provide a DEM free of pit and flat areas, without zero slope cells (Petroselli et al., 2012b). For details, see [18, 19].

Table 1. Slope Classification

Class	Slope interval(%)	Class Name
I	$S < 1$	Flat
II	$1 \geq S < 5$	Slightlysloping
III	$5 \geq S < 10$	Highlysloping
IV	$10 \geq S < 20$	Steep
V	$S > 20$	Verysteep

Table 2. Quantitative description of transformations

	Max.	Min.	Mean.	St.dev.	Area Transf. (%)	Vol. Transf. (10^6 m^3)		R	
								Area total	Area transf.
V Aniversario	453	86,5	170,5	63,43	---	---		---	---
Fill	453	86,5	170,9	63,45	4,18	15,07		0,998	0,959
TOPAZ	453	86	170,4	63,40	6,48	48,55		0,998	0,998
						-0.625	47,9		
PEM4PIT	453	86,5	179,3	57,26	47,9	1147,18		0,986	0,895

Since geomorphological changes represent a source of errors in hydrological studies based on DEM, to illustrate the degree of transformation produced by the application of the above described correction processes, the result are here analysed in terms of affected areas, elevation changes and slope redistribution. The impact on area and levation is presented as affected area and transformed volume (Table 2), some statistical description and the correlation coefficient (R) between raw DEM and corrected ones (Table 3). The R coefficient was determined for two conditions, the entire basin and the transformed area only.

About slope, it is widely known that hydrological modelling results are strongly related with the estimation of overflow behaviour, expressed by flow velocity distribution and values and the associated estimation of flow time; in many equations applied with this purpose (e.g., Darcy-Weisbach, Manning, Soil Conservation Service (SCS), Maidment et al.) the slope play a major role, and in some cases it is the only necessary parameter [19] to estimate surface velocity. On this respect, some results in literature indicate the significance of low slope areas in the hydrologic response according to [19]. In addition, since a change in elevation of just one cell could affect the slope on the eight adjacent cells during correction, slope determination seems to be the most critical step in the DEM correction process. For better understanding, we have established five class of slope, presented in Table 1, by the author [16]. The slope changes analysis will be based firstly on the presence of pits and zero slope area after corrections, which affect flow direction algorithms results. Second, the changes in class distribution, where the three first values, associated with valley bottom, seem to be highly influent in the basin hydrologic response, while class IV and V are more prone to produce velocity values out of literature velocity upper limits (2 m/s) usually adopted by models [19].

The comparison statistical methods will be explained now. Considering that the data distributions of height and slope analysed don't satisfy the conditions of normality, we carried out a comparison of paired samples, applying Wilcoxon Signed-Rank Test, to determine significant differences between the original DEM and the corrected ones, about these two parameters.

For a detailed description of the correction methods influence on the original DEM, as aforementioned we selected five class of slope, shown in the Table 1. The cells percent were compared by class in the resultant corrected DEMs according to the original.

We carry out variance analysis test (ANOVA) to determine the existence of significant differences among the transformations according the class methods.

RESULTS

Area and Volume Change

Concerning the affected area, it is possible to see from Table 2 that largest influences were produced by PEM4PIT, close to 50%. Fill and TOPAZ methods shows the less area influenced within the 5.-7% of the total area. Figure 4 shows the spatial distribution of those changes.

Keeping in mind the whole subwatershed extension the results of the correlations shows same value for the Fill and TOPAZ methods. However, when it is considered only the transformed area, the method TOPAZ shows a higher value of the correlation coefficient.

Using the Wilcoxon Signed-Rank test, we can decide whether the corresponding data population distributions are identical without assuming them to follow the normal distribution, see Table 3. As result of the Signed-Rank test, it was obtained that the Fill and TOPAZ methods don't carry out significant transformations of height inside a level of 5% significance; however, the method PEM4PIT transforms the subwatershed terrain significantly during the correction.

According to slope, the Table 4 show percent area corresponding to depressions and to zero slope. You can appreciate that three methods eliminate depressions in DEM, however, the Fill method generates an equivalent flat area to 1,56% (2,44 km^2) that didn't exist in the original DEM. As it is very well-known, this effect constitutes a deficiency, because it influences the flow direction, flow accumulation and network extraction methods, with the creation of unreal water pathways in these surfaces. The other two models don't present this result, because the small area of 0,0004% in the result of the pattern TOPAZ, corresponds to isolated cells that don't represent obstacles for the flow directions methods. On the other hand, the statistics displays the best correlation for TOPAZ in V Aniversario subwatershed. PEM4PIT inclination to affect the mean and standard deviation, however, seems to be the best for correcting regions with middle slope. We consider that TOPAZ is a fine solution for correcting flats and irregular regions, especially flats where the transformation on volume was minimal, while it could affect large area. There is an increase of 26.68 percentage points in the first class, corresponding to slopes smaller than 1%, as well as a decrease of the remaining classes, highlighting the class III with 16.97 percentage points. These results can affect the flow velocity distribution in the basin, increasing the low velocities and hence reducing the concentration time, being an error source for the hydrological models.

The Signed-Rank test for the comparison of paired samples of the slope values before and after the correction showed significant differences (See Table 3) among the slope maps of the PEM4PIT and of the original DEM.

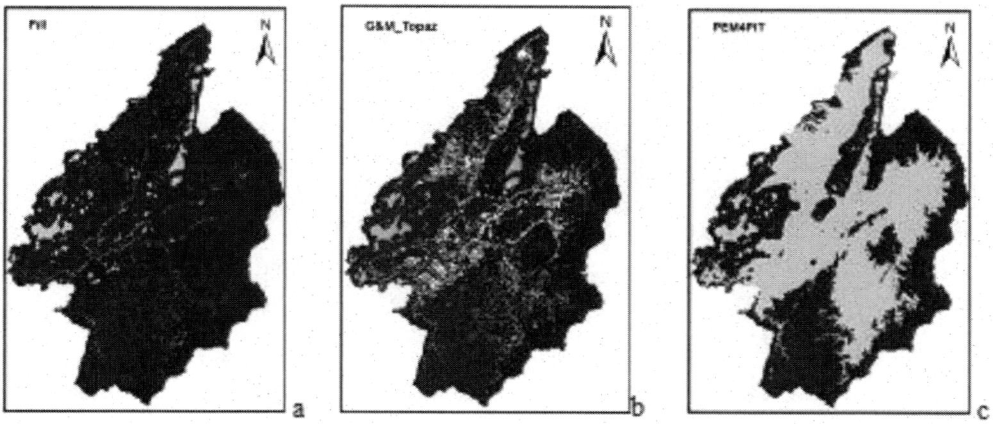

Figure 4. Maps of transformed area V Aniversario: (a) Corrected DEM minus raw DEM; (b) possitive_grey colour; (c) negative_white colour).

Tabla 3. Results of comparison of paired samples, Signed-Rank Test

Analyzed couples	P valor	
	Height	Slope
MDE Original - Fill	0,999994	0,999994
MDE Original - TOPAZ	0,999994	0,999994
MDE Original – PEM4PIT	0,0	0,0

Table 4. Qualitative description of the slope transformation

	Min	**Max**	**Mean**	**Pit(% de área)**	**Slope Zero (%)**	**Class Distribution (% regarding the total area)**				
						I	II	III	IV	V
V Aniversario	0,0063	249,44	20,28	0,59	0	3,1	19,8	16,1	23,3	37,7
Fill	0	249,44	19,56	0	1,56	4,9	19,7	15,9	23,1	36,4
TOPAZ	0	249,9	19,73	0	0,0004	4,8	19,4	15,9	23,1	36,7
PEM4PIT	0,001	249,43	15,94	0	0	29,8	17,7	6,3	14,5	31,7

In Table 5 are shown the supposition confirmation of normality and variance homogeneity, using the non parametric test of Kolmogorov-Smirnov and the Levene test, which gave as result that data are usually distributed and it presents homogeneous variances. To determine the existence of significant differences among the three groups, it was applied the test of Simple ANOVA and Duncan's Multiple Range test, in order to detect which groups differ to each other. The results show that significant differences exist among the groups, being the PEM4PIT method different significantly as respect to Fill and TOPAZ methods.

Table 5. Analysis of the class transformations

Methodo	Kolmogorov-Smirnov		Variances Homogeneity Test		Simple ANOVA Test	Duncan's Multiple Range Test		
	Estad.	Signific.	Statistical of Levene	Signific.	P-Valor	Mean	Homoge-neous groups	
Fill	0,216	0,200	2,795	0,101	0.0066	0,02088	x	
TOPAZ	0,328	0,083				0,05356	x	
PEM4PIT	0,194	0,200				0,19288		x

The results agree with the ones described by [10] about basins where there are not many plane areas: the Fill and TOPAZ methods don't present significant differences. According to the consulted literature the PEM4PIT has not been evaluated in basins with so variable relief as is the case of V Aniversario. The results could be the consequence of the significant transformations of the original relief.

About to Cuba, works have been consulted about geology and geomorphology, but from a point of view of characterization more litomorphogenetic and their time evolution. Research works similar to the present manuscript have been developed by [20] and [21] but not applied to superficial hydrology.

By way of summary we can conclude that: 1-The statistical tests expose that geometric methods (Fill and TOPAZ) are more appropriate for V Aniversario region DEM correction. 2- The method Fill carries out the correction with the smallest area and volume affectations, however, it creates a false flat area during the process, and this circumstance could constitute a source of errors in later hydrological analysis. 3- The TOPAZ method does not present this characteristic, being the more recommended for the preprocessing of the investigated case study. 4- The physically based PEM4PIT method carries out significant transformations of height and slope, so for that, its use could not be recommended for hydrological applications in V Aniversario subwatershed.

ACKNOWLEDGMENTS

The research work was conducted in the framework of the collaboration with DAFNE Department, Agrarian Viterbo Faculty, Tuscia University funded by the Italo-Latin American Institute (IILA), Italia, of which, we are very satisfying. In special, gratefulness to the researcher Salvadore Grimaldi and Andrea Petroseli, these professors have contributed in the training of the GIAF researchers.

REFERENCES

[1] Arnold, N.:"A new approach for dealing with depressions in digital elevation models when calculating flow accumulation values," *Progress in Physical Geography,* 34(6): 781–809, 2010.

[2] Jenson, S. K. and J. O. Domingue: "Extracting topographic structure from digital elevation models," *Photogramm. Engng Remote Sensing*, 54: 1593–1600, 1988.

[3] Grimaldi, S., F. Nardi, F. Di Benedetto, E. Instanbulluoglu and R. L. Bras: "A physically based method for removing pits in digital elevation models," *Adv. Water Resources*, 30: 2115-2158, 2007.

[4] Nardi F., S. Grimaldi, M. Santini, A. Petroselli and L. Ubertini: "Hydrogeomorphic properties of simulated drainage patterns using DEMs: the flat area issue," *Hydrological Sciences-Journal-des Sciences Hydrologiques,* 53(6): 1176-1192, 2008.

[5] Petroselli, A.: "LIDAR Data and Hydrological Applications at the Basin Scale," GIScience and Remote Sensing, 49(1): 139–162, DOI 10.2747/1548-1603.49.1.139, 2012.

[6] Martz, L. W. and J. GARBRECHT: "An outlet breaching algorithm for the treatment of closed depressions in a raster DEM," *Computer Geosciences,* 25: 835–844, 1999.

[7] Kenny, F., B. Matthews, K. Todd: "Routing overland flow through sinks and flats in interpolated raster terrain surfaces," *Computers and Geosciences*, 34(11): 1417-1430, 2008.

[8] Wang Y., H. Peng, P. Cui, W. Zhang, F. Qiao and C. Chen: "A New Treatment of Depression for Drainage Network Extraction Based on DEM," *J. Mt. Sci.*, 6: 311-319, 2009.

[9] Garbrecht, J. and L. W. Martz: "The assignment of drainage direction over flat surfaces in raster digital elevation models," *Journal of Hydrology,* 193: 204–213, 1997.

[10] Srivastava, A.: *Comparison of two algorithms for removing depressions and delineating flow networks from grid digital elevation models*, 255pp., Thesis (en opción al grado científico de Master of Science in Biological Systems Engineering), Virginia Polytechnic Institute and State University, Virginia, US, 2000.

[11] Muñoz, J. and Kravchenko, A.: "Deriving the optimal scale for relating topographic attributes and cover crop plant biomass. Geomorphology." 179: 197-207, 2012.

[12] Elshehaby A. "Automatic Road Network Extraction Based on Spectral Angler Mapper" International Journal of Circuits, Systems and Signal Processing, 15: 3, 2013.

[13] Fan, G. Miguez-Macho: "Potential hydrologic changes in the Amazon by the end of the 21st century and the groundwater buffer," *Environmental Researchs*, 9, ISSN 084004, 2014.

[14] Nourani and Zanardo: "Wavelet-based regularization of the extracted topographic index from high-resolution topography for hydro-geomorphic applications," Hydrological Processes, 28(3): 2, 2014.

[15] Fisher, P. and N. Tate: "Causes and consequences of error in digital elevation models," *Progress in Physical Geography*, 30(4): 467-489, 2006.

[16] Felicísimo Angel, M.: "Parametric statistical method for error detection in digital elevation models." *ISPRS Journal of Photogrammetry and Remote Sensing*, 49(4): 29-33, 1994.

[17] Petroselli, A. and A. Fernández: "The Flat-Area Issue in Digital Elevation Models and Its Consequences for Rainfall-Runoff Modelling," *GIScience and Remote Sensing,* 49(5): 711–734, DOI 10.2747/1548-1603.49.5.711, 2012.

[18] Grimaldi, S., A. Petroselli and F. Nardi.:"A Parsimonious Geomorphological Unit Hydrograph for Rainfall–Runoff Modelling in Small Ungauged Basins," *Hydrological Sciences Journal*, 57(1): 1–12 [doi:10.1080/02626667.2011.636045], 2012.

[19] Grimaldi, S., A. Petroselli, G. Alonso and F. Nardi: "Flow Time Estimation with Variable Hillslope Velocity in Ungauged Basins," *Adv. Water Resources*, 33(10): 1216–1223, 2010.

[20] Valdés F. and Molerio L.: "Hidrogeología y geomorfología cársica del Valle Ancón, Pinar del Río, Cuba." Ingeniería Hidráulica y Ambiental, 25(3): 4, 2003.

[21] Valle, R. et al.: "Caracterización Geólogo - Geomorfológica del Delta del Rio Cauto en Cuba Oriental," *X Congreso Cubano de Geología, Geología Regional y Técnica*, 2013.

In: Models and Methods for Supporting Decision-Making … ISBN: 978-1-63485-173-2
Editors: Carlos N. Bouza, Flávio L. de Mello et al.

Chapter 12

An Integer Optimization Model for Waste Collection Frequency Problem

Joanna Campbell Amos[1], Sira Allende Alonso[1] and Marcos José Negreiros Gomes[2,*]
[1]University of Havana, Havana, Cuba
[2]State University of Ceará, Ceará, Brazil

Abstract

A systematic collection service is fundamental to human health and premise for the waste recycling processes. Constraints in the availability of resources cause deficiencies in the service of solid waste collection and their accumulation in streets. In this paper an integer programming model is proposed for fixing a time table of waste collection in sectors of a given area. It is assumed known the capacity of the available collection fleet and the amount of wastes generated daily in each sector. The goal is to minimize the accumulation of waste residues in the area.

Keywords: waste collection, linear integer programming

Introduction

The term urban solid residues designs to all material that is discarded by the population, (may be domestic, commercial, industrial, public or reject of constructions) that is not considered as dangerous according to the legal framework of the country of reference.

Nowadays, waste management is one of the main environmental and social-economic problems, especially in towns and large cities which are densely populated. The rapid and constant growth in urban population led to a dramatic increase in urban solid waste

* Email: negreiro@graphvs.com.br , sira@matcom.uh.cu, joanna@matcom.uh.cu.

production. It is estimated that, the production of solid residues increase by 2 to 3% per year [7].

In populous cities the volumes of urban solid residues are significantly large. United States produces more than 168 million tons of waste annually, which represents approximatly 670 kg/inhabitants/year (1.84 kg/day). In many European countries, per capita daily waste generation is larger than a kilogram. Although significantly lower in Latin-America, the volume of waste generation exceeds capabilities for its management. For example, Brazil reached an average of 306kg/ihabitant-year by 2010 about 160 thousand tons of trash per day and in major small and average cities the residential refuse collection suffers with few available resources [10].

In Cuba it was estimated a daily generation of 4,000 tons/day of solid waste, for an average of 0.5kg per inhabitant every day. The major garbage production occurs in La Habana [2]. Equipment machining, conventional, and specialized is insufficient and does not allow an efficient service with the required quality. These resources limitations cause waste accumulation at different points of the city.

In Fortaleza city, state Ceara/Brazil, are collected more than 3,300 tons daily of waste and the Aterro Sanitário Metropolitano Oeste de Caucaia (ASMOC), which had been projected for 15 years, covered a 60.12% of its capacity in the first six years of job. Given its geographical situation, Fortaleza grows vertically with consequent increment of population density and the generation of solid waste [9].

Accumulation of waste residues causes contamination of soil, air, water. It states that 80% of diseases that affect developing countries are attributable in large part to basic needs related to environmental sanitation. It is clear that waste accumulation has a negative impact in the environment and human health, on the other side, a process of recovery and treatment which puts much of the waste in technical conditions to be returned to the market would be important from economical point of view. A project in that direction is developed in Fortaleza [8].

Some experiences on recover wastes residues have been reported in Havana, Holguin and Ciego de Avila. Studies on the composition of waste residues in Habana have reported the following results: organic matter (59.4%), paper (20.34%), metals (6.23%), plastic (1.68%), textiles (3.36%), wood (0.6%), others (7.25%) [6]. Therefore, approximately 60% of the total weight of solid waste generated is organic matter, which could be useful in the agriculture but produces odors at the points of deposit, proliferation of insects and rodents, risks of infections, production of methane and other gases.

In general, municipal authorities of all countries are forced to determine good management solid waste systems. Such a system includes optimal location of dumping sites, location of waste bins, and efficient waste collection subsystem. Some authors refer that solid waste collection services consume 30% to 60% of the municipal budget (see, for example, Karadimas et al. [7]).

Of course, it is important to fix a goof collection frequency for avoiding the waste accumulation in the streets. If available resources do not allow daily collection in all sectors, is necessary to fix rationally the collection calendar of each sector. In this paper we focus on this problem of residential waste collection frequency in urban area.

The paper is organized in four sections. The problem is described in section 2; in this section is also defined the set of possible frequencies to consider. The mathematical model is presented in section 3. A case study is discussed in section 4. Finally, we present the conclusions and future research directions.

DESCRIPTION OF THE PROBLEM

Usually, residential wastes are collected at domicile. For organizing the waste services in a region, municipalities usually consider a partition of the geographical area in sectors. The topology of the soil, population density, social and economic conditions and the activities of the sector (locations of industries, commercial, education or health centers) are taken into account for defining the sectors.

A limited vehicle fleet is available for the collection. The vehicles can differ in capacity or type (heterogeneous fleet) or not (homogeneous fleet). A vehicle is assigned for collecting the wastes of a sector according the technical characteristics of the vehicle and the requirement of the sector. The number and type of vehicles available for the collection may vary from one day to other.

The problem is to determine which days of the week should be collected the wastes of each sector for reducing waste accumulation at the street as soon as possible. It is important to precise days of the week in which each sector be served, for achieving a systematic service and avoiding unnecessary exposure of waste tanks on the streets. To decide the collection frequency of a sector it is necessary to estimate its waste generation. Municipalities have information on the weight of wastes generated in the region per habitant daily (Index of daily waste Generation per habitant, $G(s)$). Known the population of each block, it is then possible to estimate the waste generated daily by each sector, as the product of its population and $G(s)$.

Waste collection in each sector should be daily, but if it is not possible, hygienic regulations indicate that the period between two consecutive collections have to be always less or equal than two days. The goal is to fix which days of the week the wastes will be collected at each sector looking for good hygienic conditions in the region.

	Sun	Mon	Tue	Wed	Thr	Fri	Sat
F1	0	1	1	1	0	1	0
F2	0	1	0	1	1	1	0
F3	0	1	0	1	1	1	0
F4	0	1	1	1	1	0	1
F5	0	0	1	0	1	0	1
F6	0	0	1	1	1	1	1
F7	0	1	1	1	0	1	0
F8	0	0	1	0	1	0	1
F9	1	0	0	1	0	1	0
F10	0	1	0	0	1	0	1
F11	1	0	1	0	0	1	0
F12	0	1	0	1	0	0	1
F13	1	0	1	0	1	0	0
F14	1	1	1	1	1	1	1

Figure 1. Different frequencies pattern solution space.

Under the established hygienic regulations, it is possible to determine the set F of possible frequencies in the week. It leads to the construction of the *Frequency matrix* $\varphi = [\varphi_{ij}]_{f\times d}$ where each row corresponds to a possible frequency, each column to a week´s day and the elements are defined as $\varphi_{ij} = 1$ if there is collection under frequency *i* in day *j*, $\varphi_{ij} = 0$ in other case. Figure 1 shows fourteen diferrent frequency patterns, the first column corresponds to Sunday. From matrix φ it is easy to calculate, for each day *d*, the number of days transcurred from the last previous collection under each frequency *f*.

MATHEMATICAL MODEL

In this section we present a model for assignment the weekly collection frequency to each sector. It is necessary that all sectors receive the service in the week and taking in account that the sectors accumulate certain amount of wastes daily, depending of their collection frequencies. In order to ensure good hygienic conditions in the region is desirable minimizing the accumulation in the worst sector, that means, the sector with major accumulation.

We introduce the following notations:

$\boldsymbol{I = 1..m}$, set of sectors
$G(s)$: m^3 waste generated /hab/day in sector
$P(s)$: population of the sector s
$K(d)$: collection capacity in day d
φ: frequency matrix
$\pi(d, f)$: at day *d*, the number of days from the last previous collection under frequency *f*
$B(s, d, f)$: waste accumulated in sector *s* at day *d* under frequency *f*
$(B(s, d, f) = G(s) * P(s) * \pi(d, f))$

Decision Variables

$$x_{if} = \begin{cases} \mathbf{1} & \textbf{if frequency } \boldsymbol{f} \textbf{ is assigned to sector } \boldsymbol{i} \\ \mathbf{0} & \textbf{if not} \end{cases}$$

Minimize δ
Such that,

$$\sum_{f\in F} x_{sf} = 1, s \epsilon I \tag{1}$$

$$\sum_{s,f} BG(s, d, f)\, x_{sf} \leq K(d), d = 1..7 \tag{2}$$

$$\sum_{f} BG(s, d, f) x_{sf} \leq \delta, s = 1..m, d = 1..7 \tag{3}$$

$$x_{sf} \in \{0, 1\}, s = 1..m, d = 1..7 \tag{4}$$

The objective function represents the goal of reducing the total accumulation during the period. Constraints (1) guaranty that all sectors are served. Restriction on the collection capacity of the fleet is considered in constraints (2). Constraints (3) identify the sector and day with major accumulation of wastes at each collection day of the sector. And constraints (4) indicate the domain space of the decision variables.

Note that the number variables (*7m*) depends of the number of sectors and days of the week considered, but the constraints number ($8m$+7) depends of the number of sectors. Hence, it seems possible to apply this model in the practice and solve it using exact algorithms. In addition, pre-processing procedures could reduce considerably the model dimensions.

AN APPROACH TO WASTE COLLECTION FREQUENCY IN COTOROO, HABANA

In this section we discuss the possible application of the model in the context of a municipality of province Habana, Cuba, as study case.

Cotorro is a peripheral municipality of median extension with urban and rural areas. Management of waste collection services corresponds to Direction of *Servicios Comunales* of the municipality. The territory is divided in six sectors called *Zonas Comunales* (Comunal Zones) taking into account their geographical and social characteristics, five of them are considered urban areas. Vehicle fleet available for waste collection is heterogeneous and variable from day to day during the week.

The waste generation in this municipality is large, as it is shown in Table 1. In particular, zona 1 exhibits one of the major index of daily waste generation per habitant in the capital: 1.88 kg [6].

Wastes collection service is not offered at Sunday in this municipality. Hence some frequencies are excluded. Figure 2 shows the frequencies to consider to run the model avoiding Sundays. The collection fleet capacity is completely insufficient for daily collection. The fleet is very heterogeneous.

At the moment, we expect complete information about the daily collection capacity (in particular: capacity of each vehicle in kilograms and possible number of travels of certain vehicles of the fleet).

The model in this case has 50 variables and 47 constraints or 41, if we consider only six days (Sunday excluded). Hence, it is possible to solve it using an exact algorithm. To illustrate the application of the model, we have assumed a daily fleet capacity of 43,800 kg. The results are shown in table 2.

Table 1. Waste G generated /ihab./day in each zone

Comunal Zone	$G(s)$	*Population*
Zone 1	1.86	18,587
Zone 2	0.65	16,739
Zone 3	0.71	10,949
Zone 4	0.70	11,750
Zone 5	0.67	4,090

The proposed frequency satisfies the sanitary regulations and collection capacity constraints. It would be desirable a collection more frequent in zone 1, but it is only possible with a larger collection capacity or planning collection service at Sunday.

	Sun	Mon	Tue	Wed	Thr	Fri	Sat
F1	0	1	1	1	0	1	0
F2	0	1	0	1	1	1	0
F3	0	1	0	1	1	1	0
F4	0	1	1	1	1	0	1
F5	0	0	1	0	1	0	1
F6	0	0	1	1	1	1	1
F7	0	1	1	1	0	1	0
F8	0	0	1	0	1	0	1
F10	0	1	0	0	1	0	1
F12	0	1	0	1	0	0	1

Figure 2. Set of frequencies patterns considered for the instance evaluation of the model.

Table 2. Fleet scheduling obtained from the proposed model

	Mo	Tu	We	Th	Fr	Sa
Zone 1	x		x		x	
Zone 2		x		x		x
Zone 3	x		x		x	
Zone 4		x		x		x
Zone 5		x		x		x

Conclusion

The proposed model allows determining the fleet scheduling timetable for waste collection in an area. It is assumed that daily collection capacity is variable considered that collecting frequencies ensure compliance with health regulations. The optimal solution of the model allows arranging service by minimizing the amount of accumulated waste. The dimensions of the proposed model and pre-processing procedures support its use in practice. The application in real sceneries and the extensions of the model for selective collection systems are future research lines.

References

[1] Bautista J, et al. Solving an urban waste collection problem using ants heuristics. *Computers and Operations Research*, doi: 10.1016/j.cor.2007.01.029, 2009.

[2] Cardoso, M. G., C., O. and N. H, M. J. Experiencia piloto para el manejo integral de los residuos sólidos urbanos en localidades con características urbanas y semi urbanas. caso de estudio en ciudad de La Habana, Cuba. Mapping Interativo, 2009.

[3] CEPIS/OPS Análisis sectoriales de residuos sólidos en Cuba www.bvsde.paho.org/eswww/fulltext/analisis/cuba/cuba.

[4] Correa Cortés Y., R. Santos HerreroL. Gómez Moya La problemática de los residuos sólidos y su gestión en la ciudad universitaria Abel Santamaría. 2006 http://www.bibliociencias.cu/gsdl/collect/revistas/index/assoc/HASH01ea/03f3ed4f.dir/doc.pdf.

[5] Cruz, D. Gestión ambiental y sostenibilidad CEPIS REPIDISCA rep 27448, 2011.

[6] González Rodríguez Y. Territorio y Gestión de los RSU en el ejemplo de Ciudad de la Habana. Tesis de Maestría en Medio Ambiente y Desarrollo, Universidad de la Habana, 2009.

[7] Karadimas, N., Doukas, N., Kolokathi, M. and Defteraiou, G. Routing optimization heuristics algorithms for urban solid waste transportation management. *WSEAS Transactions on Computers*, 7(12), 2022-2031, 2008.

[8] Lopes de Oliveira, José Danilo; Rieradevall i Pons, Joan Reciclaje de residuos sólidos urbanos en Fortaleza (Brasil). *Revista Técnica* 14 (79) 160-8, 2004.

[9] Oliveira Gemmelle et al. Estimate of the municipal solid waste collected in Fortaleza and destined to the sanitary landfill of Caucaia (CEARÁ), 2010. web-resol.org/textos/Gemmelle-Artigo%206.pdf.

[10] Rigonatti, A., Rodrigues, J.A.V., Batista, P.L.F.B, Negreiros, M.J. Application of the Mixed Chinese Postman Problem Models and Experiences with Urban Garbage Collection: Case Study In Jardim Europa/SP, Modelación Matemática De Fenómenos Del Medio Ambiente Y La Salud Tomo 3 Chapter 4, pgs 33-45, 2014.

In: Models and Methods for Supporting Decision-Making … ISBN: 978-1-63485-173-2
Editors: Carlos N. Bouza, Flávio L. de Mello et al.

Chapter 13

Evolving an Intelligent Framework for Decision-Making Process in E-Health Systems

***Leonardo M. Gardini*[1], *Carina Oliveira*[2], *Reinaldo Braga*[2], *Ronaldo Ramos*[2], *Luiz O. M. Andrade*[3] *and Mauro Oliveira*[2,*]**

[1]State University of Ceará, Fortaleza, Brazil
[2]Federal Institute of Ceará, Fortaleza, Brazil
[3]Federal University of Ceará, Fortaleza, Brazil

Abstract

This paper presents improvements of LARIISA, a framework that makes use of context-aware information to support decision-making and governance in the public health area. More specifically, two relevant e-health applications are presented to illustrate the LARIISA system. The first one uses Bayesian networks in dengue scenarios. The second application uses ontology to manage home care scenarios. In both cases, the contributions related to the LARIISA framework include patient health diagnosis provided remotely, support for decision-making health systems, and context information for context-aware health systems.

Keywords: framework, context-awareness, ontology, decision-making, health

Introduction

Among the challenges of information management in the health area, we highlight the difficulty faced by a significant part of managers to act efficiently on decision-making

[*] Corresponding Author address. Email: mauro@ifce.edu.br.

processes. To address some of these challenges, a framework called LARIISA [1] [2] was originally conceived to support decision-making processes concerning public health governance. This framework makes use of applicable concepts such as context-awareness, ontology and personal tracking to support health managers to take more knowledgeable decisions.

This paper presents LARIISA, a framework that makes use of context-aware to support decision-making and governance in the public health area. Besides that, two applications are presented to illustrate the applicability of the LARIISA system. The first one uses Bayesian network in scenarios of dengue fever disease. The second application uses ontology to treat home care situation. In both cases, the contributions related to our framework include patient health diagnosis provided remotely, support for decision-making health systems, and context information for context-aware health systems.

This paper is organized as follows: Section II discusses shortly about context-awareness and personal tracking concepts. Section III describes the objectives of the LARIISA framework. Section IV presents the evolution of LARIISA with an intelligent model for enhancing the decision-making on the proposed system. Section V presents the two applications. Finally, Section VI concludes the paper and discusses future work.

Context-Awareness and Personal Tracking Concepts

Information could be captured revealing where the user is or what the user is doing, and then this information could be used to offer personalized services and information [3]. Context is this type of information, which characterizes a situation and can be used by decision-making processes. Applications that use this type of information are named context-aware applications [4]. Therefore, a context model defines types, names, properties and attributes of the entities involved in context-aware applications, such as users and static/mobile devices. The model attempts to predict representation, search, exchange and interoperability of context information among applications. A well-designed model is the key to any context-aware system [5].

Aiming in assisting users in their day-to-day tasks, context-aware applications have been using elements of ubiquitous systems to obtain user context information. A simple example is the use of sensors that detect the presence of people and automatically trigger lighting to an environment, according to the people location and time.

We propose the use of context information related to the user location while registering his/her remote health diagnosis. The user location is registered by using the GPS sensor of the device. The GPS coordinates and the description of the patient context are added to the patient health diagnosis, helping the decision-making process of LARIISA. The ability to track, trace and control anything from anywhere on the planet has been humankind's unfulfilled desire [6].

In this context, it can be cited Captain [7], a context-aware system based on personal tracking. The main purpose of Captain is to map the trajectory of a mobile user, adding contextual information related to each user position. The mobile application proposed on the

Captain project performs the yacht tracking, associating contextual information with each position.

While registering the trajectory followed by the mobile device, it allows users to create multimedia documents (e.g., photo, audio, video), which are connected to an enriched description of the user context (e.g., weather, location, date). Finally, all this data and documents are combined to produce a new content, which is published on the Web.

LARIISA FRAMEWORK

LARIISA defines the basic architecture for building context-aware applications and supporting decision-making in the health care area. LARIISA was specified taking into account specific requirements of five governance fields: Knowledge Management, Systemic Normative, Clinical and Epidemiological, Administrative and Shared Management [1]. LARIISA provides context-aware diagnosis based on geolocation and can be applied in different scenarios of decision-making for local and global contexts [8].

Also, LARIISA framework works with real-time information and comprises inference systems based on ontology models. It is context-oriented, providing adaptability to the decision-making applications existing in the Brazilian healthcare network. The current healthcare network is divided into five levels: Primary Care Network (also known as Family Health); specialized Ambulatory Care Network; Hospital Network; Urgency and Emergency; and Mental Health.

LARIISA system is able to perceive the status of an emergency epidemiological situation and then set up itself (in real time) to a risk situation.

Identifying which user is sending health status (enriched data) to the LARIISA Database is crucial for the proposed framework. Without this identification, it is not possible to determine who is sending health vital signs to the system. To overcome this challenge, a unique identification (ID) number needs to be informed by the user at the moment he/she starts a new health diagnosis from his/her mobile device [1]. The unique ID chosen is the SUS ID [9], an identification number assigned to every Brazilian citizen as part of the national registry of users – for the consolidation of the Sistema Único de Saúde (SUS) of Brazil [10]. In this context, the unique ID can be used to register a new health diagnosis and also query information from other databases such as SUS database, public hospital databases, etc.

We consider the use of the LifeWatch V phone, a fully featured android-based phone [11] [12]. This device has a variety of health sensors (blood glucose, body fat, stress test, etc). Our proposal is limited to the body temperature, blood pressure and heart rate sensors. It is also important to mention that context-aware systems have some dependencies that may not be satisfied in some situations. The Internet connection, for example, can be limited or even not available at certain moments. In order to minimize these dependencies, we propose some design decisions.

Data Acquisition

The Data Acquisition uses sensors available in mobile devices to get information about localization, time, heart rate, blood pressure, body temperature, local weather, etc. In addition, SUS ID and symptoms informed by the user when the application is started are also considered as Data Acquisition.

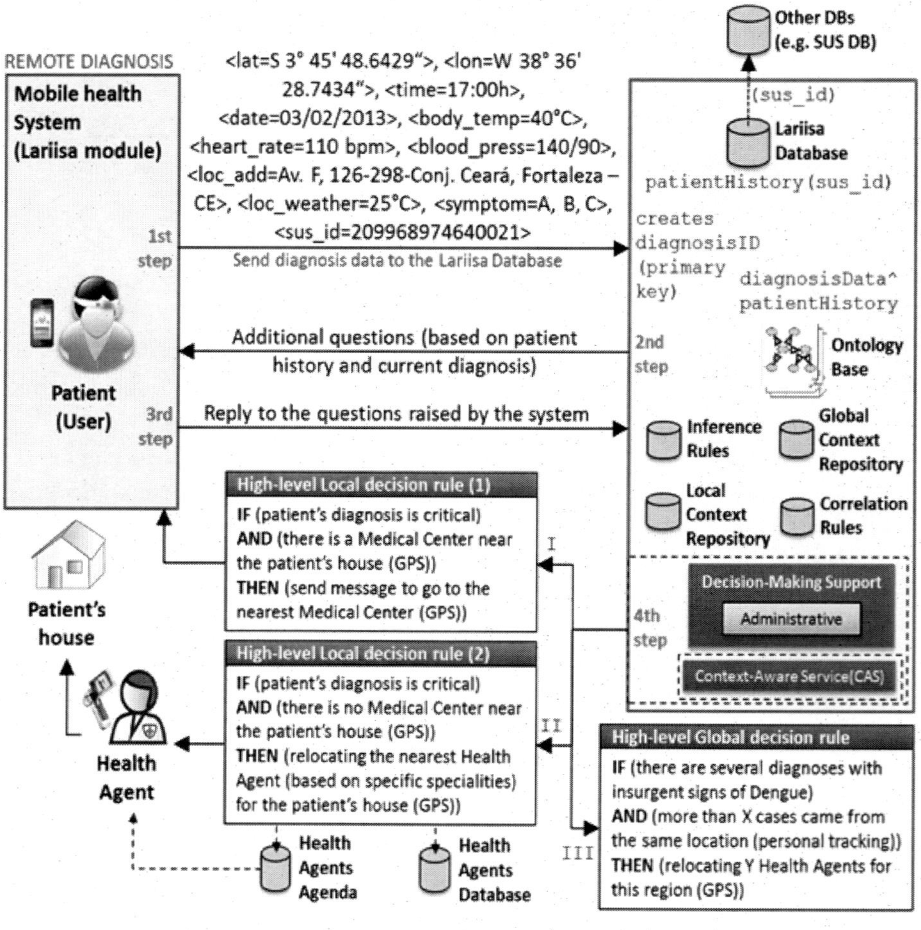

Figure 1. LARIISA Architecture.

According to Figure 1, the user starts the data acquisition process in the mobile device. After starting the application, the Data Acquisition process starts to collect all data needed to send the patient's enriched health data to the Lariisa Database. Before starting the acquisition of location, time and health, the user must inform his/her SUS ID and symptoms to the system. These data (SUS ID and symptoms) are added to the other data acquired, including health data gathered by the sensors and data gathered from the Internet via Web Services. Location name and weather can be obtained from the Internet, both using the position information acquired by the GPS. If Internet connection is not available at the moment diagnosis system is started, all data will be cached and further it will be sent to the Lariisa Database. In order to improve the Data Acquisition process, SUS ID information is stored on the system. Therefore, the user does not need to send the ID at the next time he/she uses the system.

In order to improve the data processing step, it is important to organize the acquired data into the metadata. Therefore, the system uses tags to arrange the information in the metadata.

Data Processing

The Data Processing part is responsible to increase the robustness of the system by offering more than a context-aware data collector. It associates and organizes the information in order to provide a comprehensive structure to be published (registered) on the Lariisa Database.

Making use of the acquired data organized by tags, the data processing part is started. It has to organize the data in order to facilitate the content generation for later registering on the Lariisa Database. The key idea is to use the context information of the remote health diagnosis data for decision-making support, considering both local and global contexts. The system provides enriched health diagnosis based on the information acquired by the mobile application. For example, if a user starts a remote health diagnosis, the system will generate a new diagnosis with the coordinates S 3° 45' 48.6429", W 38° 36' 28.7434" at 17:00 on 03/02/2013. Besides that, the mobile application captures health data from medical sensors (body temperature, blood pressure, heart rate, etc.), and the user is requested to add his/her health symptoms and SUS ID [9].

If the mobile device due to an absence of connection does not acquire the information of location name and weather, our system interface has to be able to obtain this information based on context information. The specialized web services provide the weather status for present and future times. To solve this problem, we propose a mechanism to capture this information using a HTML parser in order to get the location name and for the past time. This parser reads the web page DailyHistory of the WeatherUnderground and obtains the weather status related to the context information provided by the acquired data [1]. When the application generates the content to register all health status data, the third step of the proposed system can be started.

Publishing

The last part of the system is responsible for registering the content on the Lariisa Database. An important part of the architecture proposed is the use of Context Aggregator Layer (CA) to receive health status context information from context providers. This layer is also responsible for running context aggregation operations in order to have useful high-level context represented by the Local Health Context Ontology [1]. Moreover, health managers could view the content of diagnoses organized by day, by place, or by patient (e.g., filtering diagnoses results by SUS ID).

LARIISA EVOLUTION

The main characteristic of LARIISA evolution is related to our methodology for modeling the problem of pattern classification, based on patients' diagnosis data. Besides that, we consider some steps to achieve our target, which consists of analyzing the metrics in order to obtain the training set. Therefore, the training step is executed after the capture of feature vectors, which contains some sub steps, such as feature selection and the predictive labeling.

It is important to observe that the proposed pattern building and labeling approaches are independent of the chosen pattern classifiers. We emphasize that the proposed pattern building and labeling approaches are independent of the chosen pattern classifiers. The training set, i.e., the set of labeled patterns used for training is obtained through the following steps:

Step 1: Extract raw data from the database, which contains usage information of the beneficiaries;
Step 2: Perform feature selection;
Step 3: Find every patient that did a health diagnosis somewhere in the analyzed period of time.
Step 4: For each patient's diagnosis data found on Step 3, build a pattern considering a procedure window counted from the first time a target diagnosis was done. This is intentioned to capture the moment of transition when the patient passes from low risk to high risk. These patterns are called target patterns;
Step 5: Find each patient that never had a critical disease during the same time period;
Step 6: For each patient found on Step 5, build patterns considering a procedure window counted from each available month. Note that each reference month generates a distinct pattern per patient. These patterns are called non-target patterns;
Step 7: Obtain a training set formed by every target pattern and the same quantity of non-target patterns, randomly sampled.

LARIISA APPLICATIONS

In this section, two applications are described as a proof of concept of the LARIISA proposal:

LARIISA Bay

LARIISA_Bay is a component based on Bayesian networks that works together with the LARIISA framework [13]. This component is concerned with the treatment of uncertainty in health systems. Here, the representation of context-sensitive information (i.e., data collected) as well as the knowledge of experts are used [13].

As a result, LARIISA_Bay is able to assist team of specialists to better diagnose diseases according to the data collected from different users of the system.

Figure 2 illustrates the proposed phases of LARIISA_Bay. To better illustrate these phases, we describe examples of the dengue fever disease, which corresponds to the case study.

The Input System: it corresponds to an information-gathering interface that allows the interaction of three different decision makers: the patient (i.e., user of the system), the health agent and the specialist. In Figure 2, note that the specialist interface contains the health agent interface, which in turn contains the patient interface. In this initial phase, sensor can also be used, for example, to monitor patients' vital signs. As a result, metadata is created from the gathered information. It is also possible to use external context providers.

Decision Support: the Inference Module corresponds to the Bayesian network modeled to support the decision making of medical teams. The Inference Module has two main purposes in the context of the presented application:

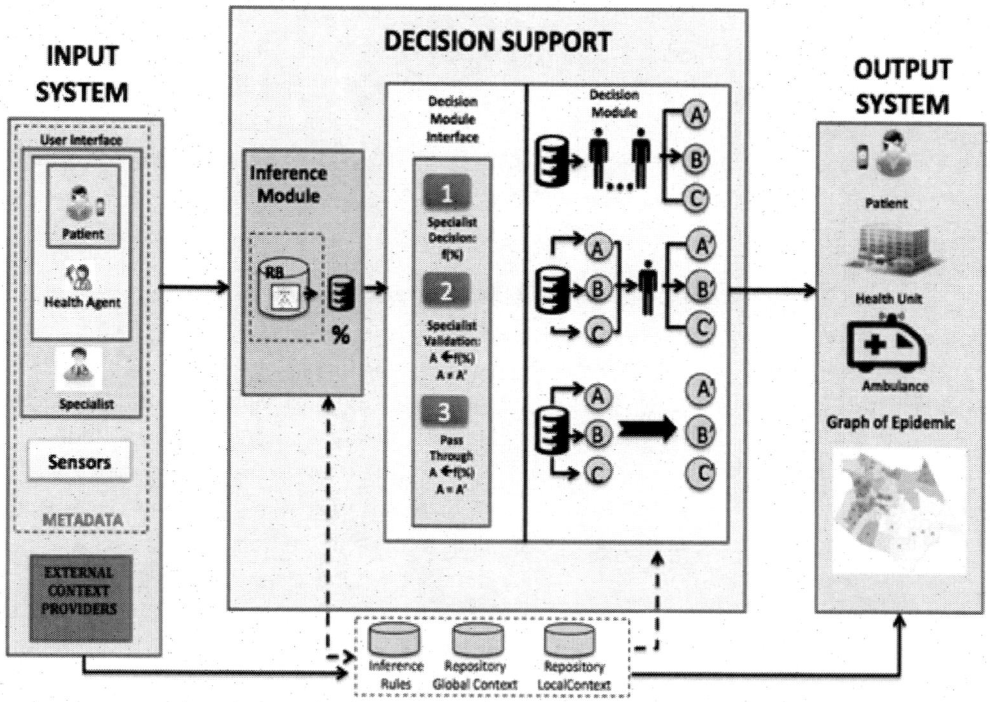

Figure 2. LARIISA_Bay Application [13].

(1) To support the diagnosis of the medical staff, filtering probable cases of dengue in three levels of classification, which are:
    i) Normal, for patients without dengue fever;
    ii) Grave, for patients with dengue fever disease;
    iii) Emergency, for patients with dengue hemorrhagic fever.
(2) To support the diagnosis of dengue fever outbreaks/epidemics in specific regions (i.e., risk areas).

Next, we have the Decision Module Interface, which offers three different application scenarios:

(1) Specialist Decision: it considers the existence of a team of experts able to better diagnose the dengue fever disease according to the received information. Based on the result of the Inference Module, the team of experts can take the most appropriate decision in relation to a particular patient;
(2) Specialist Validation: in this scenario, the result of the Inference Module is filtered/validated by an specialist, instead of analyzed, as in the Specialist Decision scenario;
(3) "Pass Through": in this scenario, one of the following decisions can be made: to leave the decision making to the system or to wait for a health specialist to take the decision.

The Output System: it corresponds to the procedures that can be made after the Decision Support phase to optimize the public health system as a whole. We can mention the following procedures as examples: send guiding procedures to the patient; send a health agent or emergency health team to the patient's home; identify risk areas (graph of the epidemic) in order to adopt proactive preventions.

LARIISA_HC

LARIISA_HC is the LARIISA's home care application. It aims to support the easy deployment of e-health applications such as services to monitoring vital signs of elderly and people with specific diseases that require medical supervision at their own home.

By allowing the usage of already deployed home devices such as the television, the system not only reduces the cost of deployment of such solutions but also facilitates the acceptability of such systems.

As shown in Figure 3, we can notice vital signs monitoring service, the physical status of patients such as temperature, heart rate, pulse, respiratory rate and also blood pressure can be displayed on the screen of the TV so that the inhabitant can easily notice any anomaly.

In addition, the LARIISA_HC provides access to communication services such as short message messaging to inform relatives of any emergency situation, programming announcements on TV reminding inhabitants of the medication time, facilitating the daily lives of elderly by reminding them important events related to their wellbeing (e.g., doctors' visits, etc).

CONCLUSION

Choosing the best mechanism to provide an accurate health diagnosis has demonstrated as being one of the main challenges to improve the whole capacity of the LARIISA framework.

We believe that an approach to overcome this challenge is to implement classifiers that choose suitable intelligent mechanism for providing the appropriate health diagnosis based on patterns and tests. Also, for some diseases the best intelligent system is the use of ontology, and for others, the best approach is the use of Bayesian networks.

As future work, we will continue to focus on improving the LARIISA framework. We plan to study the content combination of different users in order to create reference among their trajectories, personal data and contextual information.

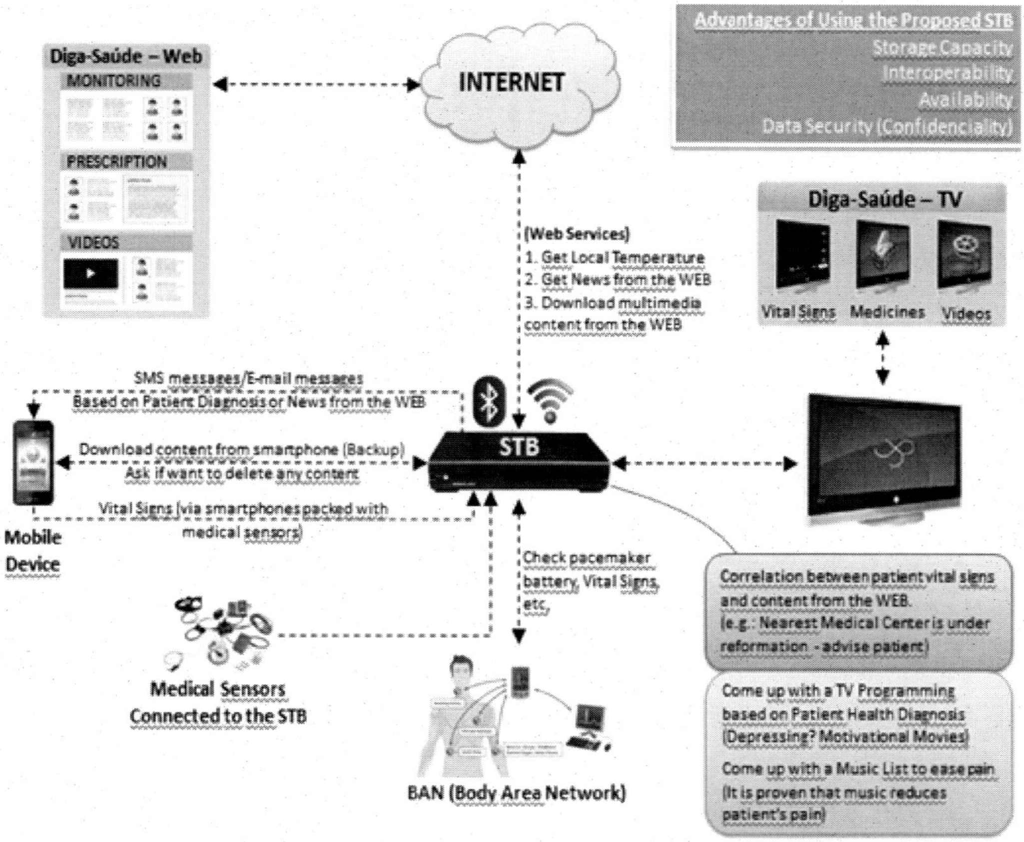

Figure 3. LARIISA_HC Application.

REFERENCES

[1] Gardini, L. M., Braga, R. B., Bringel Filho, J., Andrade, R. M. C, Oliveira, C. T., Martin, H., Andrade, O., Oliveira, M., Clariisa, a Context-Aware Framework Based on Geolocation for a Health Care Governance System. In: International Conference on e-Health Networking, Application and Services (IEEE HealthCom), 2013.

[2] Oliveira, M., Andrade O. M., Hairon C. G., Moura R. C, Fernandes S., Bringel J., Gensel J., Martin H., Sicotte C., Denis J. L. A Context-Aware Framework for Health Care Governance Decision-Making Systems: A model based on the Brazilian Digital

TV. Second IEEE Workshop on Interdisciplinary Research on E-health Services and Systems (IREHSS).

[3] Antunes F. Um Protótipo Sensível Ao Contexto Para A Governança De Sistemas De Saúde Baseado Na Tv Digital Brasileira. Master of Science Thesis on Computer Science at the State University of Ceará (Brazil), 2011.

[4] Fischer, G. Context-Aware Systems-The 'Right' Information, at the 'Right' Time, in the 'Right' Place, in the 'Right' Way, to the 'Right' Person. Advanced Visual Interfaces International Working Conference. Capri Island (Naples), Italy, 2012.

[5] Abowd, G.D., Dey, A.K., Brown, P.J., Davies, N., Smith, M., Steggles, P.: *Towards a better understanding of context and context-awareness*. In Gellersen, H.W., ed.: HUC. Volume 1707 of Lecture Notes in Computer Science., Springer (1999) 304-307.

[6] Jahnke, J. H., Bychkov, Y., Dahlem D., Kawasme, L. "Implicit, Context-Aware Computing for Health Care," http://www.ics.uci.edu/lopes/bspc04documents/Jahnke.pdf, 2004.

[7] Braga, R.B., Martin, H.: Captain: A context-aware system based on personal tracking. In: *The 17th International Conference on Distributed Multimedia Systems*/DMS 2011, Florence, Italy, KSI, 2011.

[8] Resch, B., Mittlboeck, M., Lipson, S., Welsh, M., Bers, J., Britter, R., Ratti, C., Blaschke, T. *Integrated Urban Sensing: A Geo-sensor Network for Public Health Monitoring and Beyond.* MIT Open Access Articles, 2012.

[9] Sistema Único de Saúde do Brasil, available at: http://portal.saude.gov.br/portal/saude/Gestor.

[10] Darekar, S., Chikane, A., Diwate, R., Deshmukh, A., Shinde, A.: Tracking System using GPS and GSM: Practical Approach. *International Journal of Scientific and Engineering Research.* Volume 3, Issue 5, 2012.

[11] LifeWatch V Android based healthcare smartphone packed twith medical sensors: http://www.medgadget.com/2012/07/lifewatch-v-android-based-healthcare-smartphone-packed-with-medical-sensors. html. Accessed in 05.15.2013.

[12] LifeWatch V Smartphone, available at: http://www.lifewatchv.com/. Accessed in 05.19.2013.

[13] Teles, G., Oliveira, C. T., Braga, R. B., Andrade, O., Ramos, R., Cunha, P., Oliveira, M., Using Bayesian Networks to improve the Decision-Making Process in Public Health Systems. In: I*nternational Conference on e-Health Networking, Application and Services* (IEEE HealthCom), 2014.

In: Models and Methods for Supporting Decision-Making … ISBN: 978-1-63485-173-2
Editors: Carlos N. Bouza, Flavio L. de Mello et al.

Chapter 14

HEART DISEASES PREDICTION USING DATA FROM HEALTH ASSURANCE SYSTEMS

***Ronaldo Ramos*[1,*], *César Mattos*[2], *Amauri Júnior*[1], *Ajalmar Neto*[1], *Guilherme Barreto*[2], *Helio Mazza*[3] *and Márcio Mota*[4]**

[1]Federal Institute of Ceará, Brazil
[2]Federal University of Ceará, Brazil
[3]DYAD e Associados, Brazil
[4]State University of Ceará, Brazil

ABSTRACT

Health insurance companies usually keep huge databases containing the service usage records done by their clients. In this article, we present an experimental comparison that has been made among several kinds of classifiers in order to find an optimal model to predict the development of heart diseases based on this type of data. To construct the prediction model we developed a method for pattern labeling called TWINF (Time Window into Near Future), which is used for building the test and training sets to be submitted to the classifiers. Then, over a period of four years, we conducted experiments using dozens of classifiers in order to see which one would be most suitable to forecast the occurrence of heart diseases six months earlier. Later on we will see the results of the experiments. Note that the labeled patterns used to have thousands of attributes, which lead us to a course of dimensionality problem.

Keywords: pattern recognition, data mining, cardiopathy, heart disease

---

* Corresponding Author address email: ronaldo.ramos@gmail.com.

INTRODUCTION

Several countries in the world, including Brazil, adopt private or mixed health systems. Regardless of the nature of the service, the use of medical procedures such as appointments, examinations, surgery etc. are recorded in databases and can be used for a variety of purposes including detection of epidemics, usage statistics, and even building disease forecasting models.

It has not always been easily verifiable the correlation between these data and the types of diseases that one want to detect, by the fact that, at least in this case, these are not clinical data. Undoubtedly, the lack of clinical data is a major challenge to the validity of the process, but helps us to strengthen the important fact in medicine which states that diseases usually develop as a result of the patient's behavior.

In this article, we start by showing the nature of the data we use highlighting some technical aspects of the analyzed database. Then, we show how to prepare the patterns that were used to evaluate the classifiers. In the next step, we selected a set of classifiers, present the data and verify the results. To evaluate the classifiers we have used the parameter known as Area Under the ROC Curve [1].

We found that some classifiers showed better results than others in the evaluation. That is the case of the MLP (Multi Layer Perceptron). The details of the process of constructing a prediction model are in the following sections.

THE DATABASE

The experiments were performed on a real database containing events of approximately 900k users that occurred between the years 2006 and 2011. Each record can contain up to 9031 fields that are nothing but the procedures performed by patients. In fact, the number of procedures passed the 11k, which lead us to do some attribute selection reducing them to the 9k effectively used in the inference process.

These procedures can be, for example, routine visits, blood tests, urine tests, X-rays performed, etc. In this database the set of logged events arrive at the amount of 150 million of records.

Note that is not registered in the systems the possible diagnoses or test results. We have available only the performed procedure but not its results.

At this point the main issue was to determine the classes that would be the target of our classifier. So, we selected some procedures such as coronary artery bypass surgery, heart valve exchange, transplant, stent insertion, etc. as targets procedures that categorize the record as a target, i.e., a signature of a patient with heart disease. Off course, the procedures are not all performed at once, instead, they occur over time and this is essential for the development of prediction model.

The standards of labeling mechanism are detailed in an article published recently [2], but we do a brief description in the next section for the fast understanding of the performed work.

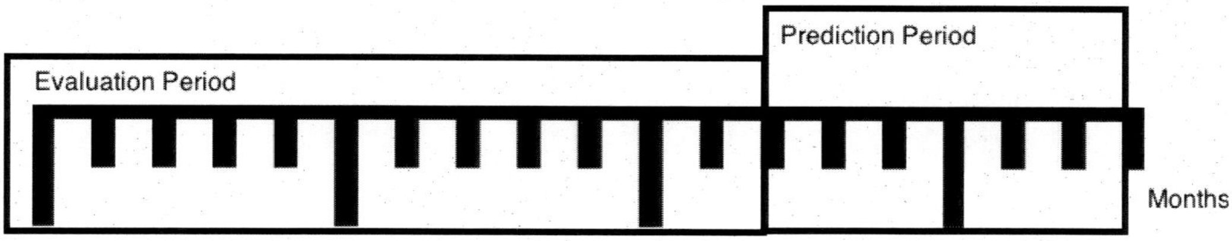

Figure 1. Time Window.

LABELING APPROACH

Initially, we have defined the timeline windows that should be used. After a few small tests with periods of 6,12, and 24 months we considered using the period of 12 months (Figure 1) to evaluation period and 6 months to the prediction period.

What happens is that the prediction period is used to label the patterns as target or non-target, and thus, build the training and testing sets on the evaluation period.

In addition to the procedures that are the features or attributes of the patterns the gender and age of the patients were added to the composition of the attribute vectors. Here we have an interference into the systems that is justified by the weight of these attributes for the detection of heart diseases. Formally, the patterns are built as follows.

A pattern P is defined as P = [a1, a2,...,ai,...,aj], where ai = 1 ∀ j ∈ [1,J-2] if procedure i was done within the time window, ai = 0 ∀ j ∈ [1,J-2] otherwise; aj-1 = 1 if beneficiary is male, aj-1 = 0 otherwise; aj = 1 if beneficiary is in a specific age group, aj = 0 otherwise. Observe that J refers to the number of attributes.

Once defined the patterns, we have performed an attribute selection procedure. The description of how the attributes are selected is also described in [2], which is basically to calculate some conditional probabilities as follows.

Let A be the event of occurrence of one target procedure (e.g., myocardial revascularization) and P(A) its probability. Let also Bj be the event of occurrence of the procedure Bj. The conditional probability P (A|Bj) is calculated by:

$$P(A|B_j) = \frac{P(A \cap B_j)}{P(B_j)}$$

The probabilities in the right side of this equation may be estimated from the examples available in our database as follows:

$$P(A|B_j) = \frac{|A \cap B_j|/N}{|B_j|/N} = \frac{|A \cap B_j|}{|B_j|},$$

where N is the total number of events and | • | denotes the cardinality operator.

Equation above is calculated for every procedure Bj. The result is the estimated probability that a beneficiary went through a target event A, given that he/she also had a procedure Bj. These conditional probabilities are sorted from greatest to lowest and only a fraction is selected. Indeed, due to the quantity of procedures, we arbitrary used only the 400 procedures with the greater conditional probability.

TRAINING PROCESS

The training set, i.e., the set of labeled patterns used for training, is obtained through the following steps:

Step 1: Extract raw data from the database, which contains usage information of the beneficiaries;

Step 2: Perform feature selection as described previously;

Step 3 Find every beneficiary that did a target procedure somewhere in the analyzed period of time;

Step 4: For each beneficiary found on Step 3, build a pattern considering a procedure window counted from the first time a target procedure was done. This is intentioned to capture the moment of transition when the beneficiary passes from low risk to high risk. These patterns are called target patterns;

Step 5: Find every beneficiary that never did a target procedure during the same time period;

Step 6: For each beneficiary found on Step 5, build patterns considering a procedure window counted from each available month. Note that each reference month generates a distinct pattern per beneficiary. These patterns are called non-target patterns;

Step 7: Obtain a training set formed by every target pattern and the same quantity of non-target patterns, randomly sampled.

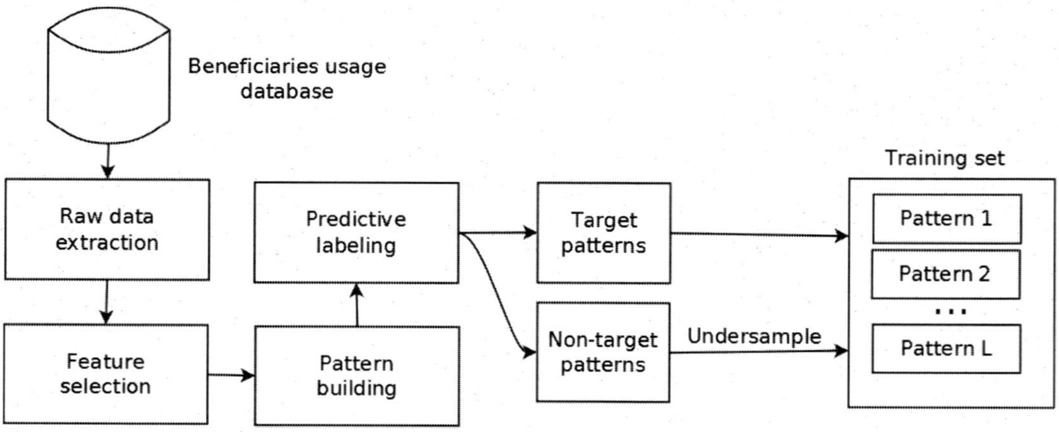

Figure 2. Composition of Training Sets.

The patterns obtained for the target cardiovascular procedures, focus of this paper, is highly imbalanced. Indeed, the ratio of target beneficiaries is close to 1:370 in our database. For tackling this kind of issue of pattern recognition, many techniques may be applied. In this study, random undersample of the majority class, i.e., the non-target patterns, was chosen during Step 7, for it is a simple and effective strategy for learning from imbalanced datasets

[3]. Figure 2 illustrates the training set building process, from the database to the feature vectors.

EVALUATIONS

Initially, we used the classical approach in order to choose the classifier that best fits the proposed model. We selected 24 data sets in pairs (training and test set) then submitted this data to over a hundred of classifiers, including some committees (such as Random Forest and Bagging). The results for some particular cases can be seen in the figures 3, 4 and 5.

Using the well-known metric called area under the ROC (Receiver Operating Characteristic) curve, we observe that the MLP (Multi Layer Perceptron) classifier (with 10 neurons in a hidden layer using unipolar sigmoid function) obtained the best results followed by KNN (K-nearest neighbours). We observed that the KNN works better, for this case, with a high number of neighbors (99 for this particular one) what appears to be an unusual value, but justified by the size of the database (900k users).

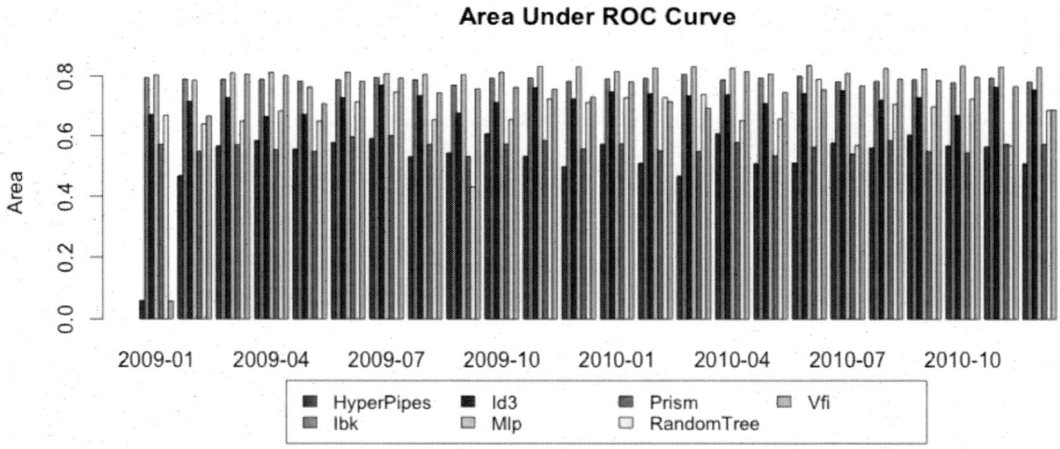

Figure 3. AUROC Comparison for Some Classifiers.

Insurance companies and users have particular interest in the prediction of all positive cases that occur in TWINF window, but are limited in terms of cost of further analysis that has to be done. Because of this, we pay particular attention to the metric recall (true positive rate) of the classifiers tested. We noted that under the recall metric, it happened an inversion between the two best (figure 4). In this case, the KNN was better for most data sets, followed by the MLP.

The problem with the classical approach is the excessive number of patterns labeled as positives. In most cases the insurer has no possibility to perform further analysis of the data collected. For instance, we may consider a number of typical data. Let's call it group 24. The test set group 24 has 621,536 entries. The MLP classifier correctly classifies 505,233 (81.28%) and therefore 116,303 (18.72%) are misclassified. Inside the subgroup erroneously classified, 115,446 (18.57%) are false positives and 857 (0.15%) are false negatives as long as in the correctly one, 1,127 (0.18%) are true positives and 504,106 (81.1%) are true negatives.

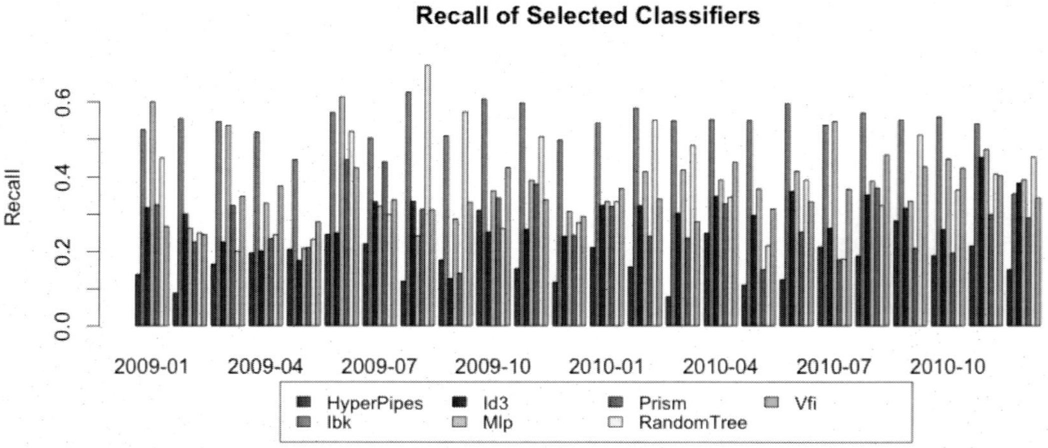

Figure 4. Recall Results for Some Classifiers.

So, we know that using the classical approach, in order to avoid 1,127 users developing severe heart diseases, we must put them, in addition to the 115,446 false positives, into a program of preventive care. Unfortunately, we can do nothing about the false negatives; however, the number of them is small.

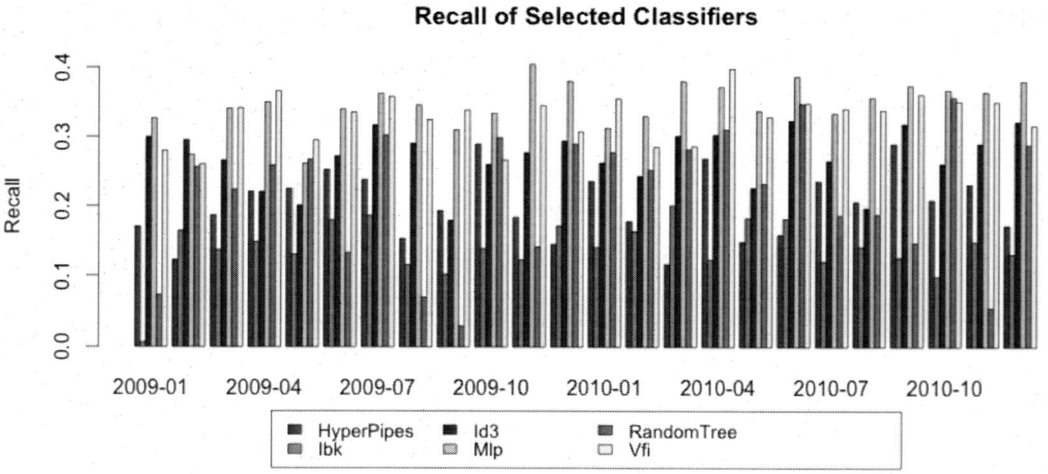

Figure 5. Recall After 5% Ranking Selection -1-24 Datasets.

Insurance companies may find that it is not feasible to submit 18% of their user base to prevention programs. The cost analysis of this feasibility is beyond the scope of this paper, but for the specific case of the company that provided the data, we have found an empirical maximum of 5%. This means that we have to limit our results to a maximum of 5% of the base. For the group 24, the number of users to be analyzed or subjected to preventive programs would be 31,077.

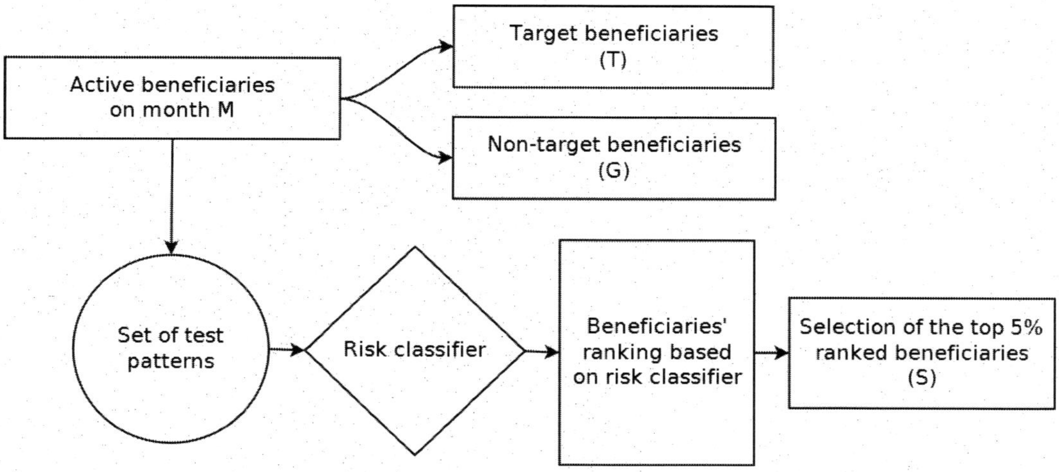

Figure 6. The Whole Evaluation Process.

To deal with this problem, we made a ranking from the information output of the classifier. The best 5% were selected. We call this 5% "sensitivity" and the application of this method has led to a slight reduction in the recall metric (Figure 5).

Figure 6 shows a diagram of the evaluation process of the risk classifier from unlabeled patterns. The steps below summarize the analysis:

Step 1 From the beneficiaries active on month M, a set of patterns is built following the methodology described in Section 2.1;

Step 2 The risk classifier previously trained receives the test set;

Step 3 The estimations output by the classifier are sorted;

Step 4 A fraction of the correspondent beneficiaries are selected. The selected beneficiaries are considered to have high risk and are, for example, sent to preventive care.

After Step 4, the recall metric may be calculated by the following equation:

$$R = \frac{|S \cap T|}{|T|},$$

where S is the set of patterns selected by the classifier as being from high risk beneficiaries, $|S \cap T|$ is the number of target beneficiaries selected, i.e., correctly identified (or true positives), and $|T|$ is the total number of target beneficiaries in the test set. For example, if the test set is known to have 100 high-risk beneficiaries and, after the application of the risk classifier, 50 of these were found, the recall would be equal to 0.5, or 50%.

Furthermore, other important metric is the fraction of beneficiaries selected in Step 4:

$$C = \frac{|S|}{|T| + |G|},$$

where |G| is the number of non-target beneficiaries in the test set. This fraction represents the sensitivity of the evaluation, i.e., the ratio of beneficiaries selected after the risk estimation done by the risk classifier. For example, if the test set consists of 1000 beneficiaries (with high or low risk) and the sensitivity is equal to 5%, the 50 beneficiaries with greater risk estimation are selected and labeled as high risk.

It is important to emphasize that the greater the recall and the less the sensitivity the better. Indeed, if the proportion of target beneficiaries is X%, the optimal (and possibly unachievable) classifier would result in 100% of recall and X% of sensitivity. Besides, there is a balance between these two metrics, for when the sensitivity is lower, the recall is also lower. As mentioned before, in this paper the sensitivity was fixed as 5% of the number of beneficiaries in the test set.

RESULTS

Table 1 summarizes the experimental results obtained with some selected classifiers. In the first column we have the name of the classifier followed in the second by the area under the ROC curve. In the third column, we have the value of recall before the final selection and besides its standard deviation. The final results are averaged from 24 datasets. Finally, we have the recall after the selection based on the sensitivity and its standard deviation.

The classifiers shown in the table 1 are: MLP, as defined in [4] (with 10 neurons hidden layer that uses a unipolar sigmoid function), HyperPipes, KNN, ID3, Prism, Random Tree and VFI.

Table 1. Summary of the Best Classifiers Evaluation

Classifier	AUROC	STD Dev.	RECALL	STD Dev.	RECALL (5%)	STD Dev.
HyperPipes	0.5243	0.1065	0.1701	0.0531	0.1985	0.0467
KNN (IBK)	**0.7907**	**0.0076**	**0.5364**	**0.0535**	**0.1387**	**0.0277**
ID3	0.7298	0.0311	0.2950	0.0699	0.2709	0.0410
MLP	**0.8166**	**0.0173**	**0.3974**	**0.1109**	**0.3464**	**0.0302**
PRISM	0.5657	0.0184	0.2806	0.0804	NA	NA
RandomTree	0.6644	0.0856	0.3795	0.1368	0.2113	0.0979
VFI	0.6967	0.1981	0.3486	0.0557	0.3285	0.0296

HyperPipes is a simple and fast algorithm. For each category one "hyperpipe" is constructed containing the points in this category. Instances are classified according to the category that accommodate or adjust the instance. It is supposed to work well on sparse data and a high number of atributes [6], which is the case here, but we only have punctual superior results. Its averaged results were inferior to the others.

The experiments with the KNN classifier presented good results when compared to the others. In fact, it achieved the best recall before the final selection. It suggests its ability to work with data of high dimensionality and sparse data. Regarding performance, the methodology used to prepare the training set assured a reduction in its size resulting in an appropriate performance (few minutes to classify more than 600k users into a Intel Core2 Duo machine).

In the experiments, we have tested several kinds of decision trees. The ID3 algorithm [5] presented results slightly lower than the MLP. It is interesting to note that it has showed just a small drop in recall after applying the ranking selection.

The Prism algorithm builds a kind of modular decision tree [7]. It has showed interesting results in a previous experiment and was chosen to be tested against these data. Note that it was ranked in the top seven.

Random Tree [8] algorithm uses a decision tree with random attributes at each node. It showed the best punctual result (0.698 recall), but remained dissimilar over different data sets.

The VFI algorithm (Voted Features Interval) [9] surprised us with good results in several moments of the research. In that case, classification is performed by votes for intervals. The intervals are constructed around the classes for each attribute. The class are counted for each attribute and then selected the most voted one.

Many other classifiers were tested with poor results, even tree-based committees such as Random Forest and also Bagging. We left as further work to set up parameters for ensembles that may improve the rates obtained so far.

CONCLUSION

In this paper, we presented a methodology to forecast the development of severe heart diseases based on historical data of patients using data available in private health assurance systems. The main point of this methodology is the pattern labeling based on future events, which forces the classifier to act as a predictor. We called this method TWINF (Time Window Into the Future).

The data are arranged in huge databases containing millions of records of procedures performed by patients from the moment of their inclusion in the health plan until their departure from it. These data were analyzed and it was found that there are thousands of procedures, which may be performed one or more time by at least one patient.

A method was proposed for each of the various steps: the selection of attributes (since it is difficult to work with arrays with thousands of rows and columns), the selection of classifiers and test execution over 24 previously selected data sets.

More than a hundred classifiers were tested against these data and the results of the top seven were shown here. We have shown the power of simple classifiers like KNN and MLP.

Furthermore, if the using of this methodology can save one life, then the undertaken research effort was afforded. It is a work of mining in a big database with some constraints about the quality of the data, as it is often not possible to guarantee the goodness of the available clinical data and previous diagnoses. The vast majority of the records referred to previous examinations and procedures performed by patients. Hence, we consider that the results meet the initial expectation of having a recall close to 50% for a sensitivity of 5%.

With the proposed methodology, we can work without the existence of the electronic patient records containing clinical data such as blood pressure, heart rate, etc. although we assume that this information could significantly increase the accuracy of the system.

As future work we imagine that we could test some committees schemes such as Stacking, Stacking C among others.

Furthermore, once we have exhausted the possibilities of using techniques of examples based learning, we will split up in two directions that depend on the company intervention in the relationship between patients and doctors. The first one would be to record the prescriptions such as diagnosis, treatment, and clinical data; a second one would be to use a human expert who could guide the process of further analysis of patients previously classified as positive by the system.

ACKNOWLEDGMENTS

The authors would like to thank FUNCAP (Fundação Cearense de Apoio ao Desenvolvimento Científico e Tecnoló gico) for the financial support.

REFERENCES

[1] T. H. Wilmshurst (1990). Signal Recovery from Noise in Electronic Instrumentation (2nd ed.). CRC Press. pp. 11 ff. ISBN 0-7503-0058-2.
[2] MATOS, C. L. C.; Guilherme Barreto; RAMOS, Ronaldo; Márcio Mota; Ajalmar Neto; Amauri Holanda. A Novel Approach for Labeling Health Insurance Data for Cardiovascular Disease Classification. In: 1st BRICS Countries Congress on Computational Intelligence/11th Brazilian Congress on Computational Intelligence, 2013, Recife. BRICS-CCI and CBIC 2013, 2013.
[3] van Hulse, J., Khoshgoftaar, T., and Napolitano, A. (2007). Experimental perspectives on learning from imbalanced data. In Proceedings of the 24th International Conference on Machine Learning (ICML'07), pages 935–942.
[4] Haykin, S. (2009). Neural networks and learning machines. Prentice Hall, 3ed edition.
[5] Quinlan, R. (1986). Induction of decision trees. *Machine Learning.* 1(1):81-106.
[6] Chakrabarti, S. a. a. (2008). Data Mining. Know it All. Morgan Kaufman, eds.
[7] Cendrowska, J. (1987). Prism: An algorithm for inducing modular rules. International.
[8] Breiman, L. (2001). Random forests. Machine learning, 45(1):5–32.
[9] Demiroz, G. and Guvenir, A. (1997). Classification by voting feature intervals. 9th European Conference on Machine Learning, 85-92.

ABOUT THE EDITORS

Carlos N. Bouza
Facultad de Matemática y Computación
Universidad de La Habana
San Lázaro y L. Vedado
La Habana Cuba CP 10400
bouza@matcom.uh.cu

Flávio L. de Mello
Electronic and Computer Engineering Department DEL/Poli/UFRJ
Federal University of Rio de Janeiro, Centro de Tecnologia, sl. H212-b
Ilha do Fundão, Rio de Janeiro, RJ, Brazil, CEP 21949-900
fmello@poli.ufrj.br

Marcos Negreiros
Mestrado Profissional em Computação Aplicada MPCOMP
State University of Ceará, Av. Dr. Silas Munguba, 1700
Campus do Itaperi, Fortaleza, CE, Brazil, CEP 60.714-903
negreiro@graphvs.com.br

INDEX

H

I

J

K

L

M

N

O

P

Q

R

S

T

U

V

W

X